Leaky Gut

Guide to Understanding the Protection

(How to Increase Your Energy and Cure Inflammation)

William Buckley

Published By **Bengion Cosalas**

William Buckley

Leaky Gut: Guide to Understanding the Protection (How to Increase Your Energy and Cure Inflammation)

ISBN   978-1-990373-75-6

No part of this guidebook shall be reproduced in any form without permission in writing from the publisher except in the case of brief quotations embodied in critical articles or reviews.

Legal & Disclaimer

The information contained in this book is not designed to replace or take the place of any form of medicine or professional medical advice. The information in this book has been provided for educational & entertainment purposes only.

The information contained in this book has been compiled from sources deemed reliable, and it is accurate to the best of the Author's knowledge; however, the Author cannot guarantee its accuracy and validity and cannot be held liable for any errors or omissions. Changes are periodically made to this book. You must consult your doctor or get professional medical advice before using any of the suggested remedies, techniques, or information in this book.

Table Of Contents

Chapter 1: What Is Leaking Digestive Tract Disorder?

When this takes place, the liver after that transforms in your immune machine for assist. It could not come as a wonder to you to find out that dripping digestive tract ailment may also additionally need to materialize itself in any type of extensive variety of strategies to your device.

It couldn't come as an unsightly surprise to you to find out that leaking digestive tract contamination need to materialize itself in any form of kind of techniques your device. While you can not name the ones "symptoms and signs," they're absolutely real fitness issues. The underlying motive of these issues want to quite properly be the visibility of leaking digestive tract sickness.

It takes some time, however in a few unspecified time within the destiny exactly what on the start modified into in reality a "intestine-barrier" trouble has honestly intensified right into cells poisoning. As properly as this therefore should cause a sequence of instances of numerous exclusive troubles. If your cells putting is endangered, microorganisms extend.

Despite the truth that your lymphatic device aims to acquire and after that lessen the consequences of these contaminants, it isn't sincerely continuously powerful. The mission is after that located on the liver and additionally the cells matrix, which have the possible to convert unstable.

Which's in which a further frame organ delves into interest, aiming to maintain a healthy and balanced equilibrium. It's your lymph system, an vital a part of your body immune tool.

The even more contaminants that input your device, the masses extra your liver labors at getting rid of them. If moreover severa contaminants accumulate, the immune machine tires itself functioning in preference to them. At the proper same time, the manner moreover exhausts your immune tool.

Leaking intestine illness happens when the lining of your gut ultimately finally ends up being indignant, bringing approximately infection. In this case, the leaks in the structure of the liner is endangered. This manner that the lining, which usually imitates a fortress wall ground permitting genuinely not something to undergo, can't do its artwork efficaciously.

Sometimes we cope with those signs and symptoms and signs as conditions. We deal with them, however do not understand why they already gift initially. The what's what is that due to the fact the contaminants to your blood keep, they in some unspecified time within the destiny have an impact on various distinct components of your bodily frame, numerous that are in spite of the fact that banding with each awesome striving to keep you healthy and balanced.

Rather, it definitely "leakages," allowing germs similarly to diverse one-of-a-kind contaminants, similarly to wholesome proteins and moreover fat that commonly aren't completely absorbed, to run away proper into your blood movement.

If as nicely hundreds of contaminants gather, the immune device tires itself laboring rather than them. At the best identical time, the approach likewise exhausts your immune device.

In the subsequent financial ruin, I speak about severa of the elements that could cause leaking gut sickness. Understanding exactly what reasons this sickness have to resource you do some thing super approximately it to accurate it.

The effects of.

Contaminant collect.

Leaking gut sickness.

As well as your liver.

If the decision issues you, you have to recognize that this some distance-too-not unusual hassle is moreover identified thru a miles greater expert-sounding call: raised digestive tract leaks inside the shape.

The lifestyles of those contaminants devices off an autoimmune reaction in which the body immune device movements your very personal cells. As nicely as this will in the long run create a set of intestinal issues, no longer the least which might be belly bloating, more gasoline, similarly to aches.

This trouble ought to basically bewilder your liver, leaving it not capable of refine every little factor successfully. When this takes place, the liver after that appears to your body immune tool for help. We have in reality presently superior that your immune remarks is nerve-racking, not capable of act as it want to.

Quickly, without a doubt the various signs and symptoms and signs and signs showing you may be experiencing adrenal exhaustion encompass: fatigue, relaxation that doesn't freshen you, loss of potential to control anxiety, hassle focusing, further to insufficient meals digestion.

Exactly what takes location whilst.

The liver is bewildered?

Numerous of these supposed symptoms and signs and symptoms display up as a desire of problems we reflect onconsideration on conditions as well as conditions in similarly to of themselves. Connecting them to leaking intestine disease isn't generally just what human beings expect of doing.

Not in truth that, however the lymph liquids for your bodily frame gather triggering lymphatic swelling. You'll speedy find out this via the usage of the visibility of swelling on your physical frame. This swelling is genuinely what creates the plethora of feasible signs and symptoms and signs and symptoms, numerous of which pass inexplicable.

Amongst the initial of your body organs impacted is your liver. The even greater contaminants that enter your machine, the a whole lot extra your liver labors at secreting them.

Since you recognize-- as a minimum as an entire terms-- just how this sickness establishes, with a piece of success you have got a higher gratitude for truly how all of the additives of your physical frame engage to assist combat contamination. Similarly, your tool collaborate to provide health and fitness. It's a two-manner avenue.

This phase of the tool is referred to as intestine-associated lymphatic cells, or GALT. These cells lie inside the lining of the digestion system and furthermore inside the intestinal tract mucous.

An extra body organ after that eventually ends up being impacted with the aid of the usage of this overrun of germs. Your adrenal glandulars, 2 little glandulars resting atop each of your kidneys, are essential in withstanding infection. The extended visibility of dripping digestive tract disease in a few unspecified time inside the future-- and furthermore little by little-- lowers the healthy and balanced characteristic of those glandulars.

If your very first concept is that there couldn't possibly be a health and fitness hassle called dripping digestive tract disease (LGS), it's far honestly low-value. Allow me guarantee you that, no matter the allopathic clinical area's rejection to recognize leaking digestive tract, masses of all-natural fitness treatment specialists are very aware of it.

- Yeast contamination.

- Persistent anxiety.

- Environmental contaminants.

- Persistent irregularity.

- Nutritional shortages.

- Food diploma of sensitivities.

- Extreme consumption of subtle components.

- Autoimmune contamination.

- Reduced- fiber weight loss plan.

- Low-stomach acid.

- Particular drug remedies.

- Liquor usage.

- Serious burns.

As the disorder proceeds unabated, cortisol tiers waft down. As well as it sincerely is at the same time as a hassle known as adrenal fatigue takes vicinity.

The germs after that boom to undesirable tiers, and moreover this unlocks for opportunistic infections to show up. These are infections you commonly might probably now not set up. Because of the significantly damaged u . S . Of your body immune device, they "slip in.".

Get inside the.

Lymph machine.

It deftly collaborates the feedbacks of numerous sports activities of severa frame organs inside the direction of your device. If for any form of difficulty the equilibrium is disrupted, the damaging chemical materials as well as some physical debris reap furnished to right into exactly what is known as the cells matrix.

Just how LGS exposes itself.

In your fitness and well-being.

You ought to ask your self why the frame immune tool is impacted. It's an unexpected reality (and moreover currently one you're aware about) that 70 percentage of your body immune tool is in fact positioned spherical your digestion system.

Chapter 2: The Reasons For Leaky Intestine Disorder No Person Speak About

NSAIDs in addition to.

Prostaglandins.

You mean my Candida albicans.

Could be created with the useful resource of.

Leaking gut infection?

Yes! If you have were given truely ever earlier than dealt with a Candida albicans contamination after which you recognize first-hand exactly what the u . S . A . Of dysbiosis looks like. A minimum of 1 kind of inequality.

Obviously, you understand your physical frame a extremely good deal higher in comparison to every body else. You understand your health and fitness practices. And additionally geared up with this intimate info, at the same time as you exist with a tick list of feasible covert motives you can have the capability to divide one of the most viable property to begin with and moreover look at them out.

By this moment, you would in all likelihood have presently started out an all-natural properly being expert or a naturopathic doctor that thinks that you might possibly virtually have dripping gut illness. Certainly, your immediately reaction became probably, "Exactly what created it?".

The initials constitute nonsteroidal anti inflammatory medicinal drugs. The time period differentiates this direction of drug from steroids, that have similar anti inflammatory impacts at the bodily body. All the NSAIDs are furnished as over-the-counter medicine, without the requirement for a doctor's prescription.

If this fragile equilibrium is disrupted, the Candida albicans capitalize with the useful aid of growing and furthermore overwhelming particular places of your digestive system device. Their lifestyles is going fairly a touch bit similarly in evaluation to that. These fungis produce a chemical called acid protease, which "takes" the secretory IgA from the mucous membrane layers.

The medical vicinity has in truth been counting on this just remarkable type of medicinal drug for actually concerning each state of affairs you could do not forget. The majority of people nearly require some kind of prescription antibiotics when they walk proper proper into a health practitioner's administrative center grumbling of a disorder, additionally inside the event that they do not revel in from a microbial contamination.

If you are looking ahead for your nicely being treatment industrial enterprise employer accessible over one supply on a silver plate-- well, fail to keep in mind concerning it. Generally locating the supply is in some instances one of the maximum very tough component of coping with the sickness.

For numerous people, it likewise suggests that once they really revel in pain, they choice it prolonged long long past as fast as feasible.

That's the element several people immediately get to for a course of discomfort drug treatments normally understood via its initials, NSAID.

A host of logo-new research laboratory screening and additionally matching research have a look at produced a resurgence for the situation.

Not honestly that, however extended utilization of NSAIDs will growth your threat of making abscess of the stomach and also the duodenum.

This little amount is effortlessly maintained below manage many way on your tremendous vegetation (you probably presumed that presently!) alongside aspect a sturdy body immune gadget and moreover a properly balanced intestinal tract pH.

The detrimental toll they will be taking on your bodily frame isn't in truth recounted rapid. Eventually they will cause chronic troubles, numerous which in no way ever acquire detected.

Anti-biotics help to beautify my properly-being. They heal my infections-- all varieties of infections. Well, you obtain the idea.

When this equilibrium is interrupted in addition to your bodily frame consists of masses greater negative in comparison to awesome microorganisms, this state is called dysbiosis. It's stemmed from the phrase cooperation, which suggests "staying in consistency" similarly to the prefix dys because of this that "not.".

Exactly what's the utmost purpose of dysbiosis? The stepped forward usage of NSAIDs is just one cause to the advancement of the assemble-up of awful germs.

Offered the u . S . Of modern-day-day remedy on the flip of the 20th century, this stood for an notable leap beforehand within the remedy of microbial infections.

When you area prescription antibiotics to your physical body, you are possibly interrupting the equilibrium of digestive tract germs. They cast off the lousy microorganisms-- the ones developing your situation-- similarly for your nice flora.

The overrun of germs places the liner of your bowels in threat. The in all likelihood repercussion? The manufacturing of a large desire of possibly unstable tablets, collectively with 2nd bile acids, amines, phenols ammonia, indoles, in addition to hydrogen sulfide.

Below are simply some of the loads more standard motives for this illness:.

Dr. Metchnikoff exposed the herbal microorganisms of yogurt have to avoid in addition to in reality reverse microbial infections. Not certainly that, but many manner to his have a examine, he uncovered that the microorganisms in yogurt has the capability to displace many microorganisms which generate contamination. Furthermore, the yogurt germs fabric could possibly furthermore lower the amount of getting into conjunction with contaminants.

The digestive gadget repair works.

Itself each 3 days!

NSAIDs as a purpose.

Consequently, those materials want to damage your digestive lining with the resource of way of harming the comb obstacles. The brush limitations are the most crucial maker of digestive device enzymes on your tiny intestinal tract. At some point the harmed brush barriers enzymes is probably taken in right into your blood motion.

One of the most commonplace microorganism to show up as a result of this inequality is the yeast contamination Yeast, a fungi.

The big bulk of Americans rely upon the ones medicinal tablets as a way to resource relieve all kinds of ache, from a migraine to persistent joint infection. Few human beings, but, offer any kind of actual concept to their possible negative outcomes. The development of leaking digestive tract sickness is amongst them.

We stay in a way of life that surely requires delight principle. To some human beings, that shows heaping big quantity of moneys of leisure on themselves.

They're demanded with restoration in addition to solving your physical frame! When you take an NSAID, you truely are obstructing the pain and moreover imparting to your very personal lots-wanted remedy.

Furthermore, NSAID utilization must bring about colitis and moreover regressions of ulcerative colitis. That understood that the and not using a trouble available, almost common drugs every person takes with not often a doubt may be so in all likelihood bothersome?

You might also need to appearance just how the expanded usage of NSAIDs obstructs the preferred repair company way.-- you have were given dripping gut illness.

Enormous microorganisms.

As properly as your well being!

With the advent of prescription antibiotics and moreover booster photographs, however, his take a look at seemed a bargain lesser similarly to ... Properly, pretty without problem, obsoleted. Till nowadays, this is!

That's! Despite their jobs, but, the over-the-counter remedy indiscriminately obstructs all the transmitters.

Dysbiosis.

Desire heaps more desires to reduce your reliance on them? This direction of medication creates blood loss, damages to the mucous membrane layers of your bowels, and moreover intestinal swelling.

- Misuse of liquor.

- Persistent anxiety.

- HELP.

- Candida fungus.

- Dysbiosis.

- Persistent usage of NSAIDs.

- Injury.

- Absence of Secretory IgA.

- Endotoxins.

- Intestinal contamination.

- Cancer cells remedy.

- Body immune system overload.

- Aging.

- Environmental contaminants.

- Diet recurring.

- Persistent infections.

The success of NSAIDs depend upon their capability to impede little organizations called prostaglandins. These pills distribute in the course of your physical frame and furthermore block pain similarly to swelling. The activity of those drug treatments does now not end there.

Yeast contamination is a fungi that almost anybody comes with about with them. Normally your device truly includes little portions, no longer enough to stimulate an contamination.

Those anti-biotics.

That gain me properly?

The sturdy grip of.

Yeast infection.

Because of this, your system can be observed out to immune microorganisms (individuals who prescription antibiotics can not seem to cast off effectively), fungis, bloodsuckers, and moreover infections. Typically, a healthy nicely balanced gut may want to preserve this type of trespassers away, many way to the visibility of great plants.

You're presently acquainted with the ought to keep an equilibrium in among the dangerous or pathogenic microorganisms-- as they are contacted the clinical neighborhood-- similarly to the useful germs, often known as flora.

If you resemble me, you have got were given truly probably in no manner ever turn out to be aware about dysbiosis. The word become produced via Dr. Eli Metchnikoff, a 1908 Nobel praise victor for his paintings with awesome microbial plant life.

When the equilibrium turns closer to the an entire lot extra volatile microorganisms, the effects may be irritation, swelling further to, furnished ok time, the visibility of situation.

Clinical scientific studies is finding microorganisms that do not belong in the digestion device. These germs need to moreover be a useful aid of toxin to you.

When top notch anti-biotics.

Spoil!

And moreover this permits the Yeast contamination to regular proper into and also ultimately continuously boom on your mucous membrane layer. Currently the infection is strongly installed!

If that had no longer been lousy enough, at the same time as secured similarly to strongly in feature, the Candida albicans leakages contaminants that (once more, you're an movement earlier of me) leakage right into the blood drift. When dispensing within the direction of your physical frame, the contaminants not clearly dispirit your body immune gadget, but they moreover play chaos with the hormone equilibrium of your gadget or perhaps interrupt the wholesome and balanced everyday normal overall performance of your human mind!

So there had been a honest one- or -phrase reaction to that inquiry, however there isn't always in reality. There are a gaggle of feasible motives of this disorder. And also there are "hid" triggers that severa do now not also appear to talk about.

Just what is following?

Just how round raised food stage of sensitivity?

Ways to inform if.

You have a Candida fungus contamination.

Prescription antibiotics after that generally react with the useful resource of signaling your immune machine to the visibility of unique food which in turn complements your diploma of sensitivity to those food. Later on in this financial ruin we are going to move over the difference in amongst meals stage of sensitivity in addition to a actual meals allergy.

Lots of humans get this contamination through the prolonged usage of anti-biotics further to steroid drug treatments. Lots of girls create it with the proceeded usage of contraceptive pill. As properly as even though others discover that the intake of liquor have to activate this problem.

Exactly how are you going to grow to be privy to a Yeast infection? Could you be walking round with one proper presently without moreover information it?

Steroid pills.

And moreover dripping digestive tract disorder.

Given, any shape of amongst the ones signs and symptoms and symptoms ought to show numerous other underlying contamination similarly to the visibility of a yeast contamination. Which's exactly why Yeast may be tough to discover-- in addition to goes undetected for as extended.

They're dependable on severa continual final fitness issues as well as persistent fitness and properly being issues. Long time period utilization of steroids, however, in some unspecified time inside the destiny deteriorates your immune tool. As nicely as really, you presently recognize this can create problem.

The remaining component you require is to be informed that these real same pills might be sparking the improvement of leaking gut disease. As well as which means you can in some unspecified time inside the destiny get a trouble with taking in ingredients.

It's like kicking an man or woman while he is currently down. You're managing robust most cancers cells treatment drug remedies thru radiation remedy.

This isn't truely simply supposition. The disturbance of this carefully tuned equilibrium is in truth properly recorded in clinical literary works.

Your depressed immune machine permits for the boom of a fungus infection, no longer honestly to your intestinal tool, however in really concerning every severa different factor of your physical frame.

- Unclear thoughts.

- Persistent vaginal infections.

- Level of sensitivities to the placing.

- Frequent bladder infections.

- Stomach bloating.

- State of thoughts swings.

- Irregularity or Looseness of the bowels (or every!).

- Food degree of sensitivities.

- Sleep issues.

- Reduced blood sugar level.

- Exhaustion.

- Premenstrual illness.

- Stress and anxiety.

- Anxiety.

- Ringing inside the ears.

Discuss.

Negative results!

Obtained tension?

Believe dripping digestive tract sickness!

One of the maximum volatile component of meals allergic reactions is the pretty rapid response your bodily body has. Often instances it takes region internal mins, which indicates you have to not simply understand the selection with the irritant without delay, but prepare to behave unexpectedly.

Do I truely have.

A meals degree of sensitivity?

It holds real, continual anxiety impacts your frame immune machine-- and moreover besides the a wonderful deal better. It dispirits your capability fight infections collectively with slowing down the healing approach of injuries in addition to accidents. When beneath tension, your physical body lowers its production of secretory IgA and moreover DHEA, an adrenal hormonal agent that postpones the aging manner as well as aids you manage anxiety.

This, therefore, triggers acidosis within your cells and additionally the swelling of cells further to cells.

Your physical frame perspectives the ones food bits as global compounds, which indicates your immune machine to spring right into hobby. At the suitable identical time, the liver responds.

Prescription antibiotics after that usually react with the aid of manner of warning your immune device to the visibility of unique ingredients which in flip increases your degree of sensitivity to those components. Later on on this bankruptcy we can talk approximately the difference in among food degree of sensitivity as well as a actual food hypersensitivity. Did your leaking digestive tract sickness cause your meals degree of sensitivities? Or did your meals diploma of sensitivities set off the dripping intestine sickness? Numerous people perplex meals stage of sensitivity with a actual food allergic reaction.

Too tons anxiety moreover slows down the digestive tool way, decreases blood circulate to your digestive device frame organs and moreover in the long run gives to the production of risky metabolites. Metabolites, with the resource of the way, are compounds critical for your metabolic rate.

Did your dripping intestine ailment create your food level of sensitivities? Or did your food degree of sensitivities activate the dripping digestive tract ailment? Something is alternatively specific: each appear to move collectively.

Because tension is lots a issue of our lives, I sincerely have actually committed a whole bankruptcy to numerous strategies that might help you as it should be address the tension to your life. This financial ruin on my own can be crucial to assisting you decorate your dripping gut sickness.

Your healthy eating plan as a useful beneficial aid.

Of leaking gut disorder!

People are touchy to any form of kind of components, but the adhering to belongings represent truly 80 percentage of the dangerous responses: beef, citrus end result, milk items, eggs, beef, and moreover wheat.

When you continuously consume those factors, you truely boom the leaks within the shape of your guts. A vicious cycle after that creates, because of the fact you may virtually advantage loads extra food level of sensitivities frequently.

Possibly you do not forget your fitness and properly being hassle-- or several troubles-- is created finally through your leaking intestinal tract lining. Your following step is to look a physician that thinks that this illness in fact already exists. She or he can also need to run you with a battery of analysis examinations to exactly establish your fame.

Allow's start with food hypersensitive reactions, as you're probably plenty greater accustomed with them. An hypersensitive reaction to peanuts stimulates an instant response within the bodily frame.

When the setting.

Strikes you!

Some human beings revel in an entire lot more extreme outcomes: breathing distress, the shutting your throat, bronchial allergies, or maybe anaphylactic wonder.

Several people perplex meals degree of sensitivity with a real meals allergy. There's no time similar to the existing to speak about the variations.

It's time to have a look at one supply of leaking intestine ailment over that you have manage. I will now not dive deeply right into this case proper proper proper here, due to the fact that I absolutely have truely dedicated a whole financial wreck to rebalancing your machine with adjustments on your ingesting workout routines.

Among the initial repercussions of this situation is the damaging down of your connective cells. Not extended after that, your bodily frame starts offevolved doing not have in specific trace element like calcium, potassium, in addition to magnesium.

Among the problems with the American weight-reduction plan recurring is its unique absence of fiber. When you eat a weight loss program regimen that lacks fiber, you are effectively advertising an prolonged transportation time-- a situation it surely is not for correct meals digestion.

Not just that, however the signs and symptoms and symptoms and signs and symptoms run the variety, makings the quantity of sensitivity difficult to widely diagnosed.

Some all-herbal health experts and furthermore conservationists u . S . A . You could probable be subjected to severa circle of relatives poisonous irritants, unstable chemical substances, ecological chemical substances, similarly to poisonous steels every day.

You, as properly, are impacted every day ... Hr with the aid of hr ... Also min via the usage of min ... By the putting. I'm speakme regarding a few massive negative impacts that might probably be hurting your bodily body additionally as you evaluation this.

Make fantastic to check out the financial disaster on rebalancing your machine collectively with your weight loss plan. It'll beneficial aid hobby marvels in restoration your dripping digestive tract ailment.

The difference in between.

Food degree of sensitivity as well as hypersensitive reaction.

A level of sensitivity takes area even as the food bits run away with the harmed mucosal membrane layers, stepping into right away proper into the blood circulate.

Food allergies, moreover understood as kind 1 or prompt contamination response, spark off the comments of unique a selected type IgE antibody. This antibody bonds to the meals antigens which after that launch compounds called cytokines.

The preliminary characteristic of a food level of sensitivity is that clearly generally the effects of it aren't proper away evident. This exhibits up in its clinical name postponed infection reaction.

What form of examinations? Follow me to the subsequent monetary damage and additionally I'll tell you.

Chapter 3: Identifying Leaking Digestive Tract Disorder

There's likewise a third hazard. Your exam exposes reduced tiers of each of the sugar particles.

The exam isn't genuinely very difficult or made complex to do. The results will surely expose your tiers. You'll furthermore gain facts on finding out the effects effectively.

Begin through starting a healthcare expert you rely on similarly to that comprehends the improvement of leaking gut disorder.

If the exam suggests the boom of dripping digestive tract contamination, you will preference to adopt a number of plenty extra examinations, a number of which search for more than one severa exceptional properly being troubles.

There's even extra. (It may be very a bendy examination, presently proper?) This useful exam likewise gauges your degree of a pancreatic enzyme referred to as cholecystokinin and moreover the quantity of brief-chain fats, in addition to the diploma of butyric acid for your colon.

At the workplace.

Or in the residence?

One of these examinations is called an intensive digestive system feces evaluation. Not simply that, however the examination assesses the general country of your digestion nicely-being.

If you pick out now not to test out a clinical scientific health practitioner to adopt this examination, a house package deal deal deal is with out a problem available. You definitely adhere to the recommendations and furthermore ship it off to a pre-pre-specific laboratory for evaluation.

Is dysbiosis.

Existing?

It moreover motives the pancreatic to create enzymes, both of which are critical for suitable food digestion. Butyric acid assists with developing your metabolic way, regulating swelling further to helping you address tension.

The CDSA is likewise a useful device in moreover greater strategies. (Why ought to not you be bowled over by way of manner of this?) It furthermore determines the condition of severa digestion competencies, along with the food digestion of wholesome proteins, fats, and additionally carbs.

To be absolutely precise, you ought to think about obtaining an entire scientific evaluation. That's all well further to notable. Merely wherein do you begin?

Lots of laboratories will in fact furthermore include guidelines on numerous varieties of treatment-- which includes the choices of drug remedies and furthermore all-herbal answers to recover you to a wholesome and balanced digestion degree.

Remarkably, severa people with a excessive lactulose diploma and moreover a reduced mannitol-- that is the chance of dripping gut ailment-- likewise experience Gastric contamination (the dearth of potential to soak up gluten in wheat and also numerous other items), Crohn's situation, and additionally ulcerative colitis.

Beginning to assume dripping intestine contamination exists at the end of your precise health trouble? Are numerous of those signs and symptoms and signs further to problems-- from Candida albicans yeast infections to food diploma of sensitivities-- seeming familiar?

It likewise does a beneficial 1/3 feature. It establishes the life-- in addition to viable diploma-- of Yeast in your gadget. If you don't forget the lifestyles of this fungus contamination is cautiously related to dripping digestive tract sickness.

If this yeast infection exists, your health-care employer will without a doubt take a society to set up the amount of cash of improvement in addition to to turn out to be aware about an approach for treating it.

In a healthful and balanced digestive tool method, the cells soak up mannitol outcomes. On the numerous different hand, the lactulose definitely absorbs in part. The outcomes of this exam ought to signify a excessive diploma of mannitol and also a reduced degree of lactulose for a digestion device that isn't in truth impeded via dripping digestive tract illness.

In spite of those apparently unpronounceable names, the concern definitely isn't always truely all that made complicated.

The preliminary motion in identifying the trouble is challenge a lactulose-mannitol examination. You may additionally want to furthermore pay attention this examination called the PolyetheGlycol Examination or PEG.

If the other holds proper-- reduced mannitol in addition to immoderate lactulose-- it shows the visibility of leaking digestive tract illness.

Examining wherefore?

Bloodsuckers?

Simply an eye constant fixed the listed proper right here similarly to you may see especially definitely what I endorse. These are a number of the signs of the visibility of those little animals.

Along with each weight-reduction plan regimens, there are moreover multiple blood examinations which could in all likelihood be rapid finished to useful useful resource discover degree of sensitivities. These project through gauging your physical body's reaction to antibodies. These unique equal examinations are moreover useful for food allergies similarly to level of sensitivities to ecological problems.

That's specifically why the lifestyles of bloodsuckers is so hard to find out. Extremely usually, bloodsuckers normally aren't additionally taken into consideration as a motive of any of those signs and symptoms.

Physicians after that provide you a dental laxative causing looseness of the bowels, which presses the bloodsucker along the device further to out, so it does appear for your feces if it exists.

Some medical examiners absolutely pass the feces example and also as an opportunity rent a rectal swab.

Lots of all-herbal nicely being experts need to supply you with screening on this global. Determining the precise food or chemical substances intensifying your device ought to seriously boom your possibilities of healing your health and nicely-being problem.

- Rest issues.

- Coughing.

- Anxiety.

- Belly pain.

- Gas.

- Damaged Body immune device.

- Bloating.

- Inexplicable weight reduction.

- Pearly whites Grinding.

- Itchiness.

- Unusual immoderate temperatures.

- Discomfort.

- Anemia.

- Bloody feces.

- Joint discomfort.

- Muscle mass pains.

- Breakouts.

Essentially, you can in no way ever recognize you have got got were given a parasite residing off of you. If you pay hobby very carefully to your physical frame, it's miles presenting you diffused suggestions. Refined, in truth, that they could all as well brief be disregarded or also incorrect for signs of various super nicely-being troubles.

Lots of bloodsuckers usually are not sticking around to your reduced bowels similarly to will not turn up in an arbitrary feces instance. Several are rather located further up alongside your digestion tool. In the ones instances, feces screening could in fact reveal an negative very last outcomes.

Naturally, to acquire one of the maximum actual medical evaluation is to begin a laboratory specializing in parasitology screening.

The visibility of bloodsuckers has sincerely stronger significantly for severa factors. Infected water products, the beautify in addition to comfort of global touring, the improvement in preschool with loads of youngsters touching with each severa distinctive similarly to discussing playthings, and additionally dwelling inside the direction of our home dog puppies are surely the various numerous possible factors for the developing bloodsucker populace.

There are 2 strategies of screening for those: a elimination food regimen recurring and also a justification food regimen recurring. I'll communicate even greater concerning healing with those techniques in a later chapter.

You'll require to discover a laboratory that checks mainly for IgG or IgG4 antibodies. Some laboratories furthermore embody screening for IgA, IgE, and additionally IgM.

Whew! Anything else.

I actually have to build up examined?

Bloodsuckers do not seem incredibly appealing, yet it's miles a fact: about one in 6 people brings as a minimum one bloodsucker, baseding at the Centers for Condition Control. This is most probably the fine this amount has without a doubt ever earlier than been.

Yes! An greater examination.

For food level of sensitivities.

Some natural fitness clinical professionals exam for bloodsuckers-- likewise called parasitology screening-- using arbitrary feces examples. In a few instances the examination calls for to be finished some of instances preceding to any type of straight forward clinical prognosis may be made.

Random feces.

Examples?

Yes, we are now not as an possibility performed! There are numerous even greater examinations to make sure a very precise clinical analysis, no less than if you expect you have got any form of degree of sensitivities to food or chemical substances. As you apprehend, those are 2 signs and symptoms and signs and symptoms which you could probably experiencing leaking gut illness.

These are all examinations that require to be carried out with the useful aid of your physician. You would likely likewise gain a turning healthy eating plan everyday technique in addition to severa special literary works on the state of affairs.

One very last examination!

Can you believe you studied it?

Precise clinical analysis:.

Not a critical hassle.

Your doctor may also endorse one final exam. This determines the functionality of your liver to put off contaminants. Several herbal fitness and health experts do that with the beneficial aid of offering you a caffeine pill laptop, a ache killers, and additionally 2 acetaminophen tablet computer structures.

Lots of human beings should probable preference to stay one motion in advance further to start making some of an appropriate changes in their way of existence and additionally sports speedy. Interested and additionally irritating to smooth your bodily body of this hassle?

Some all-herbal health and well-being health workers examination for bloodsuckers-- moreover called parasitology screening-- using arbitrary feces examples. In enhancement to the 2 diet plans, there are likewise a couple of blood examinations which can be effects accomplished to help display degree of sensitivities. These unique same examinations are moreover valuable for food allergic reactions and additionally stage of sensitivities to ecological problems.

As you could see, precisely detecting this disorder isn't a number one difficulty. If you consider that a right scientific diagnosis have to useful resource alleviate numerous unassociated conditions and also gather you sincerely feeling nicely over again, it is actually well actually properly well worth the initiative.

You would possibly probable moreover pay interest this examination referred to as the PolyetheGlycol Examination or PEG. The consequences of this exam ought to display a immoderate degree of mannitol as well as a reduced degree of lactulose for a digestion machine that is not really avoided via way of dripping intestine illness.

When you obtain your medical assessment, your scientific professional will really deliver you with a software program program of remedy. The adhering to bankruptcy consists of a number of the goods he's going to probable speak with you.

Each of those is cleansed with the aid of a outstanding direction of the liver. Transformed right into metabolic via-merchandise, those substances must after that be decided with a pee instance.

Chapter 4: Rebalancing The Digestive Gadget

System Hear.

Your Physical frame.

I recognize you can discover how you could remodel wearing occasions-- further to stay with them!-- in addition to lease a few nutritional nutritional supplements to useful resource growth the device. You'll take a look at fixing your digestive gadget and also previous to you recognize it, you may get at the roadway to recuperation!

Also previous to you start altering your diet regime, you can take an clean movement. It consists of eating your meals. A lot parents devour not genuinely as nicely quick, however furthermore as properly difficult.

As nicely as expect it or otherwise, moreover using hormonal stores may want to damage healthful and balanced microorganisms, as may additionally want to the consumption of steroids. Wow! Currently you may see exactly how speedy a digestion device could be broken!

You need to take the primary actions with a way referred to as reseeding the digestive tract. This is a term Frank Lipman uses in his ebook known as, Overall Revival: 7 Secret Pointers to Strength, Vigor similarly to Long-Term Health and well-being.

Presenting:.

The removal diet plan.

You're likewise possibly information simply how this disease, which isn't regularly referred to in allopathic medical circles, is probably adverse your tool extra than you at the beginning understood.

One greater thriller to acquiring nicely is following your specific requirements. Recently, you could have overlooked your bodily body even because it aimed to tell you a few difficulty come to be incorrect. Or possibly you've got surely aimed to pay interest, however now not diagnosed in reality what it modified into claiming.

The very fine steering is to stay clean of these substances for at the least four to six months. (I apprehend you can try this!) If you have got numerous meals allergies, you'll likely preference to significantly consider a turning diet regime.

Look at precisely what we as a manner of life are calling wholesome fee. Great sorrow, we have "sensitive cheese food" quantities which may be speculated to fill in real cheese, liquids at junk food consuming establishments that do not grow to be aware about themselves as milkshake or smoothies (so mainly just what are they crafted from?), and additionally a few taco meat that isn't truely One Hundred Percent red meat.

In numerous strategies, this indicates of eating is genuinely now not anything even more in contrast to a hassle manipulate device. Exactly how numerous of your friends tough work forty plus hrs every week (every

Mommy in addition to Father), riding pressure children to bop commands, football in addition to that recognizes in fact what else?

You could have been experiencing dripping digestive tract ailment for a long term currently-- probably lots longer in contrast to you could image. Your digestion device will not be recovered over night-- in addition to not additionally in a difficulty of an afternoon or 2. If you are decided out to gain nicely, you'll.

It's a straightforward diet regime theoretically; not so clean to perform. The frantic way of living of the ordinary American-- in addition to absolute confidence you could advise this to your existence-- is that there commonly aren't good enough hrs in the day. Much frequently, you likely eat junk food, ingesting hooked up order robust, as well as clean-to-put together packaged substances.

It furthermore shows as an awful lot as be a sincerely sly state of affairs. While you're worrying treating it as one hassle, it proceeds to boom even worse.

As detail of your.

New way of residing.

You're likewise thinking if something can be finished to enhance the situation. Dripping digestive tract illness seems at the least a vicious cycle you're punished to cope with.

Loosen up whilst you eat. The range of dishes have you ever ever ever consumed just currently which have been fast eaten in an automobile or downed unexpectedly preceding to you took thing in a vital conference? Most likely greater than you want confess.

Boosting the floor room implies that your digestion gadget will now not should feature so hard. The spit generated on the equal time as you eat holds digestive tool enzymes that during truth launch the approach of food digestion on every the carbs and moreover the fat.

And moreover you have were given a fuller information of truely what your actual health and properly-being issues are. This implies you'll be plenty plenty extra attuned to the suggestions your bodily frame is sending you.

The preliminary consists of any type of food allergies you could have. Any form of meals hypersensitive reactions or moreover food diploma of sensitivities (which might be moreover an lousy lot greater difficult to discover in contrast to hypersensitive reactions) need to no longer be omitted.

These three pinnacle traits are ensured to help you recover from this trouble. Prior to I additionally talk regarding the changes to your healthy dietweight-reduction plan as well as any shape of nutritional dietary supplements you require to be taking, I truely have truely given you with multiple pointers others have really made use of successfully.

I'm travelling allow you in a thriller most people normally are not informed approximately: eating your meals is essential due to the truth that it enhances the location of the food. Does no longer seem like a big offer, does it?

Prescription antibiotics are the sizeable supply. While they may be definitely valuable with the useful resource of removing the microorganisms triggering infections and moreover infection, at the same time as doing just so they moreover exterminate a segment of your superb germs.

While this could seem difficult similarly to tough, it actually isn't always actually. It includes enhancing useful germs and moreover cells in your physical frame. Beneficial germs are commonly described as probiotics.

Fortunately is that leaking digestive tract sickness will be healed. And moreover the even-higher records is that it may be executed without using difficult, possibly destructive as well as volatile tablets.

Every doctor informs you the ideal equal factor: eating is the preliminary step to a healthful and balanced digestion device.

Among one of the most desired method of bring once more equilibrium is through reworking your ingesting behaviors. Several humans make use of variations of truely what's called the elimination weight-reduction plan routine to take care of meals hypersensitive reactions, further to particularly meals stage of sensitivities, which an awful lot regularly are the underlying deliver of leaking digestive tract disorder.

That implies you are truly chargeable for the dominion of your fitness and nicely being. Recuperating from this problem is absolutely in your hands. I absolutely have in reality acquired masses of self-self assure in you.

Any sort of type of sports activities damages your machine's supply of probiotics, which consist of consuming way an excessive amount of processed meals, the ones nutritionally vacant treats. Additionally, healthy and balanced germs might be ruined through using a few tablets.

Glandulars referred to as parotid glandulars, located below your tongue, deliver messages now not actually for your digestion device, but your human mind. They tell them precisely what to expect. If you do not consume efficaciously, you seize them with the aid of way of surprise.

Persistence. Determination.

Determination.

A fast.

Beginner's brief guide.

Up formerly, you've got got sincerely been analyzing extra about the motives for leaking gut illness. You have without a doubt additionally uncovered that identifying the trouble with any kind of precision is not actually a completely smooth (or fast) hobby!

Lots of people whose allopathic physicians do not acknowledge this problem wants to live with it. That isn't always in reality always the situation. It does now not advocate you need to.

Unlike prescription antibiotics, which take away the damaging germs, probiotics in truth offer your bodily frame with a wealth of healthy and balanced or quality germs that hold your machine strolling effectively in addition to infections and additionally contaminants in exam.

The pessimism of.

Anti-biotics.

Below's genuinely.

one phrase of caution.

You're likely encountering lots of modifications in your way of lifestyles even as it problems your diet regime ordinary-- at the least in case you're appreciably tackling this sickness.

Is it any type of marvel your digestion tool is resisting?

You'll likewise be asked on any form of removal eating regimen ordinary to give up polished sugar, satisfactory-tuned white flour, in addition to grains collectively with gluten. These, as nicely, should play mayhem together along side your digestion device.

It likewise lets in you to provide your bodily body some of the precise nutrients that the packaged, delicate, and moreover junk meals do not have. In among those 2 factors, you will start to definitely revel in some distance better.

Kick sensitive meals.

To the cultured!

This technique of meals screening offers a - fold manner. By doing away with severa of the worst wrongdoers for as a minimum a month, you're permitting your bodily body to rebalance. Because time, you may be presenting it with some of the vitamins similarly to probiotics to supply lower lower back a correct bacteria-vegetation share.

As aspect of a removal healthy eating plan, the ones substances need to be the very first to be ... Properly, completed away with. Chockfull of factors similarly to weird colourings, they may be pretty commonly the most lousy culprits.

This isn't to say you can in no manner ever consume a person of those food once more. You'll positioned components lower again proper into your gadget grade by grade, maximum likely one meals at a time. You have a take a look at your physical frame's feedback.

Drawback symptoms and symptoms and symptoms?

Allow's chat vegetables and fruits.

As a whole.

You'll likewise intend to comply with multiple sincere requirements. One of the most vital movements are to eat a low-carbohydrate weight loss plan routine similarly to stay clean of sugar, liquor, and moreover vinegar.

Basically, the greens and fruit easy is precisely virtually what it looks as if. You consume without a doubt easy vegetables and cease end result for 7 to ten days. You ought to furthermore make use of olive and moreover canola oils as spices all through this time round.

While I will now not enter into any kind of facts regarding a selected diet regime in this bankruptcy, the appendix has an example of a three-segment removal diet plan that might provide you some perception of simply how this labors.

Past that, as an person that endures with leaking intestine disease, those recovery compounds need to have furthermore masses greater implying for you.

While the not unusual turning healthy dietweight-reduction plan typically encourages a four-day turning approach, you could discover that an extended period is vital for a few components.

One of the most normal substances which prompt allergies encompass wheat, corn, citrus stop end result, vegetables, in addition to cow's milk.

While you are changing your healthy eating plan, you will in all likelihood furthermore intend to reinforce similarly to increase the results by using taking dietary dietary dietary supplements. They can also want to assist encompass a strike on your numerous extraordinary tasks.

- Asparagus.

- Garlic.

- Wheat.

- Red onions.

- Bananas.

- Jerusalem artichoke.

- Barley.

- Chicory.

- Burdock.

- Leeks.

- Fruit.

- Soybeans.

They may additionally want to offer any form of form of natural strategies to promote this. One of the most inexperienced of those consist of using garlic, oil of oregano tablets, grapefruit seed essence, mathake tea, berberine, capryllic acid, pau d'arco, further to tanalbit.

If you are some of the ones human beings, after that you may take "infant movements" to start the manner shifting. As brief as you begin doing this, you could choose that you could discourage for your own off the salt-laden packaged further to froze ingredients complete of artificial elements. Think me, any sort of motion you are taking in the direction of solving your healthy eating plan will without a doubt beneficial resource.

One green method to cope with drawback signs and symptoms is to eat water, weakened fruit juices, and moreover decaffeinated natural teas. This speeds up the removal of contaminants.

You'll furthermore preference to include using a pinnacle great probiotic item. As fast as you "decorate" your gadget, the protected vegetation now not just help to repair your equilibrium, but truly give up the development of the terrible microorganisms.

Take into interest the.

Turning diet regime.

These foods are enormously endowed with compounds known as anti-oxidants. They're attributed with helping to maintain you from putting in such troubles as volatile as coronary heart infection and additionally maximum cancers cells. Anti-oxidants likewise beneficial aid to enhance your immune machine.

Some specialists assert that a person complimentary radical should probable detrimentally have an effect on one million cells. The particular amount of cash of damages superior, however, relies on the capability of your bodily frame to discover exactly what's taking region to it-- then, surely, the accessibility of antioxidant nutrients to war them.

Below's a phrase of warning. Numerous human beings begin to definitely sense even worse preceding to they really enjoy plenty better. Your physical frame has in reality extended relying on masses of those meals-- especially polished sugar!

What? You're now not obtaining your everyday call for of FOS elements.

Additionally, you can desire to start handling the visibility of any shape of Candida fungus yeast infection. This fungi without a doubt reacts properly to now not simply dietary changes, however to treatment with all-natural drugs.

Among the perimeters of Yeast contamination is their inherent impulse of survival. You need to find that still while you faithfully cope with your Candida fungus infections with probiotics, a few yeast remains stubbornly retaining straight away to you. In order to put off your device considerably, you will probable want to make use of severa fantastic strategies to make certain the contamination is prolonged beyond.

As stated, masses of human beings find out that month of abstaining from the ones culprits suffices to rebalance and furthermore restore. For a few people, but, it may use up to three months previous to any type of conclusive consequences can be seen.

For novices, it quits the extension of any shape of growth of developing food hypersensitive reactions. While there are a few food which might be lots greater appreciably diagnosed to reason a sensitive reaction, truely concerning any form of meals, if ate up as nicely commonly, have to encourage an allergy.

To be dependable, they want to be made use of as a crew. Anti-oxidants are placed in severa fruits and additionally greens, so it's far truely no surprise that so severa fitness specialists endorse these meals.

When you eat wholesome proteins further to meats, bypass slight at the red meat further to pork. If in any manner viable suppose natural meats similarly to definitely loose array chicks. Not genuinely are the ones ingredients greater healthy for you, but you'll find out that they have a actually plenty higher preference compared to just what you have surely been consuming!

Precisely definitely what meals are we speakme regarding? All versions of this weight-reduction plan regimen are sincerely comparable.

As in any kind of cleaning habitual, you may experience ache the very first some of days.

Numerous humans file they installation migraines. This signs and symptom may show up for any kind of range of factors, which include sugar or caffeine downside.

One greater word of care: as you deal with your fungus infection, it'd accentuate. Do no longer panic.

Just what is even extra, the enhancement of probiotics goes a extended method inside the course of improving your frame immune device.

Discover the benefits of.

FOS meals?

Each day, impossible sorts of cells are damages through precise debris known as complimentary radicals. Often you'll listen to the ones described as responsive oxygen kinds, or ROS.

You do not additionally understand clearly what FOS is or really what it does? The majority of human beings are sincerely uninformed of those substances and furthermore of FOS in positive.

Along with vegetables and culmination, full-size assets of anti-oxidants encompass nuts and also seeds. The what's what is that a number of food, if consumed of their natural country, have lively anti-oxidants. As fast as we refine those food thru cold them or making use of them in packaged and moreover delicate meals, we take away their normal performance.

Operating in show.

Comply with multiple.

Straightforward necessities.

This is definitely one extra signal that the cleansing way is functioning. You should relieve the situation thru vapor bathrooms, saunas, in addition to furthermore rubbing your skin with a loofa or a clean certainly dry brush.

Include smooth veggies and fruit juices after 10 days. These are unbelievably powerful further to focused property of vitamins which your physical body have to rent brief. Juices furthermore have the advantage of having the functionality to decorate detoxing paths, baseding on Elizabeth LIpski, writer of guide, Leaky Digestive tract Disorder.

Your bodily frame generates those tablets commonly as a response to metabolic technique. They are likewise generated in diverse special way. They increase swiftly while you're taking in liquor even as you are subjected to cigarettes, radiation, medicinal capsules, in addition to stinky oil.

You'll encompass substances back right into your gadget often, maximum possibly one meals at a time. While there are some food which might be plenty more considerably identified to cause a sensitive response, simply regarding any kind of meals, if fed on additionally typically, may also need to cue an allergy. When we refine those meals thru cold them or using them in packaged and additionally touchy substances, we dispose of their overall performance.

The tremendous balancing act of ...

Microorganisms.

Striking the downside signs and symptoms ...

Conveniently.

You may additionally want to have an actual passion in it quick, at the same time as you discover precisely how it can useful aid rebalance your digestion system and moreover ease the signs of dripping intestine ailment.

Do you sincerely apprehend genuinely what anti-oxidants are in addition to definitely how they tough work on your system? To in reality price their fee, you have to apprehend precisely what they do.

Prior to we speak about this smooth, allow me warn you that any shape of amendment in healthy dietweight-reduction plan-- in particular one this is predicated upon a fine category of elements particularly-- want to be removed along with your individual scientific medical doctor. They has a laboring know-how of honestly what form of changes your physical body may want to address.

Holding decrease back those meals out of your system may additionally moreover need to generate short-term terrible responses. When you surpass those signs and symptoms, despite the fact that, you'll enjoy all of the advantages which can be vowed via this approach.

These truly loose radicals are essentially unpredictable particles searching out protection (that may condemn them?). They look for electrons similarly to nab them on their non-public. And additionally they uncommitted in which they accumulate them!

That's no longer the best approach they amplify-- further to boom unexpectedly. Direct publicity to the sunlight hours likewise triggers a upward push their improvement price in addition to topics your physical body to anxiety.

The turning weight loss plan is an wonderful technique of preserving your food allergic reactions beneath control. Generally, you devour naturally applicable meals on the precise same day.

Several people would possibly find out delving into amongst those weight loss program plans intimidating. Others ought to surely discover it tough to transport "cold turkey" from packaged as well as diffused factors.

Have you cleaned.

Your device these days?

Raise your consumption of these foods in addition to you'll be helping to rebalance your digestion machine.

The food ample in this particle embody:.

Now, you are most in all likelihood beginning to gain a enjoy of simply how your physical frame operates in consistency with the factors you deliver it to preserve it strolling in important type.

While this happens in each person, the lifestyles of rate-unfastened radicals is lots greater risky whilst your digestive machine is harmed. Now, they take vicinity in such big numbers that your system cannot manage them.

You ought to likewise find out that psyllium seeds or newly ground flaxseeds aid. Begin with one tsp of both of these in water after that consume suddenly previous to it transforms proper right into a gel.

These are clearly crucial necessities to attain you all started on changing your diet plan to beneficial resource get higher your health trouble. Do now not mark down the overall ordinary overall performance of taking any form of movement-- no issue exactly how tiny.

Certain, your mommy most in all likelihood had this speak with you currently as she pleased after you the importance of vegetables and cease bring about your diet habitual. This time we are beginning the priority from a exceptionally diverse perspective.

Hooray for.

Anti-oxidants!

Utilizing this healthy dietweight-reduction plan ordinary, you may in truth devour the meals you've got got a mild or borderline response to, on the identical time as decreasing the signs and symptoms. Some human beings choose to take a look at force the turning healthy dietweight-reduction plan previous to they delve right into a removal weight loss plan.

These unstable compounds commonly purpose your mobile in addition to mitochondrial membrane layers, together along with your peripheral nervous gadget.

They might also want to negatively impact your enzymes, also. This is mainly risky because of the reality that enzymes are accuseded of making sure healthy and balanced mobile function.

Interested concerning which is probably the very excellent? Count on the following bankruptcy. I'll provide you some suggestions regarding the very pleasant nutritional dietary supplements to accumulate you began out.

That's now not all. They furthermore have the viable to break your DNA, that is the framework identifying the technique which your cells reproduction.

FOS technique a truely lengthy word, fructooligosaccharide. (I knowledgeable you it modified into long!) This is a customized type of sugar particle which in reality boosts the development of vegetation-- especially lactobacillus, a specially wonderful flowers.

Among the feature symptoms and signs of leaking intestine illness is the manage of awful germs over fantastic flowers. In rebalancing your inequality, you could most probably preference to rent the help of your man or woman scientific professional or an all-natural healthcare service.

Any shape of food hypersensitive reactions or moreover food degree of sensitivities (which might be additionally plenty extra tough to find out in comparison to hypersensitive reactions) ought to not be neglected. Much as nicely commonly, you most in all likelihood eat speedy food, dining popularity quo take out, and also smooth-to-prepare packaged ingredients.

As nicely as that is exactly the motive a few experts that deal with dripping intestine illness recommend a greens and fruit cleaning. It's not absolutely an efficient method of cleaning, but it's miles moreover slight on your tool.

Do now not permit that save you you. The honest truth which you're experiencing drawback signs and signs and symptoms suggests that the purifying is functioning. Contaminants are being removed of your machine.

Chapter 5: Rebalancing With Nutritional Supplements

It surely is a family event even as it concerns the B-complex of nutrients. As properly as due to the dysbiosis that is an herbal thing of dripping gut disease, the own family people is under hearth.

Considering its overarching significance in the health and well-being of those that enjoy dripping gut sickness, you could intend to significantly consider taking a glutamine supplement. You ought to buy this in severa sorts. You preference to look for a supplement large l-glutamine.

Vitamin A.

To get better leaking digestive tract!

Vitamin C's effective.

Antioxidant capacities!

Vitamin An activates the producing of protection antibodies understood as SigA. Furthermore, this acquainted nutrient additionally assists in the maintenance of your digestive tract mucosa.

Prior to supplementing your system with this vitamins, you can intend to ask your medical professional to run primary blood examinations to look in case you're reduced in B-12. He or she have to discover the right method that will help you reconstruct your tool.

The meals enough on this compound embody beans, beef, beats, cabbage, chicken, milk devices and furthermore fish.

Exactly what forms of nutritional dietary supplements am I talking regarding? This financial break materials you with a choice in which to choose out. You're positive to discover no much less than one that assists you in treating your dripping digestive tract illness.

Glutamine.

If there were ever before a "superhero" of the food regimen globe, it'd in fact be nutrients C. It has truely lengthy been known as an inexperienced immune booster. Countless people take it continually at some stage in cool and moreover influenza length.

It is critical you try this considering that, collectively with the the rest of the nutrient own family, B-12 is crucial in an appropriate overall performance of your nerve system.

The accessibility of severa styles of diet A are severa from fitness meals establishments, nutrition shops, similarly to moreover grocery shop institutions. You may want to desire to search for a specific sort of this vital nicely-being form block. And additionally it can be taken without any form of tension of poor side results in quantities of 20,000 to twenty-five,000 IU every day.

When you rebalance your digestion device, you can every decrease the quantity of nutritional supplements you are taking, or in any other case take any kind of in anyway! At the minimum, that need to be your goal.

For those elements, your physical body calls for a charitable amount of glutamine for the repair art work and also renovation of a healthy and balanced tiny digestive lining.

It's additionally important for you, as one that endures from leaking gut sickness, for a further problem. It's the physical frame's "endorsed strength" for the cells which line the mucosa of your tiny bowel. These particular cells employ glutamine immediately instead of expecting the blood movement to deliver them.

It is to be had in each a pill or as a powder. The advocated offering for any individual whose symptoms and signs and signs and signs and signs and symptoms and signs are modest to severe is in amongst 5 and moreover 20 grams each day.

For the equal antique person, a vitamins B-12 scarcity is notably uncommon. The physical frame shops severa years' sincerely worth making sure you stay healthy and balanced. For people with leaking gut, your physical body cannot get proper of access to the stores and also the nutrient is of no usage.

They may be determined in the kind of nutritional as well as nutritional dietary supplements. While the best shape of obtaining your vitamins, minerals, further to anti-oxidants is in fact thru whole, sparkling substances, the discrepancy to your machine might require more resource.

That's in which those first rate dietary will increase been to be had in. They ought to provide you without a doubt the precise quantity of the preferred basis to useful resource fight a dangerous trouble this is been enabled to rest to your digestion machine for furthermore extended.

That's common with dripping digestive tract. Its trademark signs and symptom, as we've got really claimed occasionally, is the barring of the absorption of severa nutrients.

It's B-12 that specially is intimidated via using the usage of this inequality of microorganisms for your tiny intestinal tracts. And also consequently, you may set up-- along facet your leaking digestive tract issues-- negative anemia. Destructive anemia takes region even as you physical frame is doing no longer have in Vitamin B-12, although it's manifestly getting the ideal deliver thru nutritional property further to dietary supplements.

It's a family people occasion!

Vitamin B complex.

Possibly one of the maximum important amino acid in the maintenance of each the framework and moreover the function of the bowel, glutamine is important for a wholesome and balanced metabolic fee. It may be gotten generally with masses of excessive-protein meals.

An extra interest appointed to this amino acid is the avoidance of the translocation of microorganisms from the digestive tract right into the blood motion-- an critical element to restoration dripping gut illness.

Possibly you have certainly additionally commenced out on multiple moves in the path of that purpose. There are various distinctive movements you may take to increase those adjustments.

The tremendous strategies to accumulate extra.

Glutamine.

2 incredible elements already current-day why it's miles a complement really worth taking in case you enjoy from this problem. And additionally nutrition C is a effective antioxidant!

Although you is probably consuming all of the excellent foods, mainly when you have genuinely started your removal weight loss plan, think about supplementing your weight-reduction plan ordinary with this effective resource of healing.

Much greater in comparison to that, the immune-boosting power of this weight loss program need to assist get higher this problem.

Do now not undervalue.

Vitamin E.

An more well-known powerful anti-oxidant, vitamins E probable locations 2nd surely to nutrients C in its effectiveness. Its location of specialised as an anti-oxidant is recuperation cells from free-radical damages. Like food plan C, it likewise has unbelievable immune-boosting powers.

Some fitness and well being specialists advise as loads as four,500 mg of nutrition C ordinary. Occasionally taking big quantity of moneys of vitamins C may additionally need to backfire on you further to purpose digestive system issues.

Baseding at the Workplace of Dietary Supplements, a adult might also want to safely take 1,000 mg a day. You may also want to mean to begin regularly, however, so your bodily body might also need to comply to the nutrient.

Exactly what concerning magnesium?

This degree of dietary supplements aids improve your body immune tool. Any form of providing surpassing this in truth has a harmful have an effect on for your immune device.

Vitamin E.

Another regarded one extra well-knownEffective anti-oxidant E probable ranks probably fees 2d honestly C in its usefulness.

Current have a observe discloses that for folks who cope with both Crohn's contamination further to dripping digestive tract, zinc dietary supplements genuinely recovers the final fitness and properly being problem. As nicely as that during turn can also want to relieve or get better Crohn's contamination.

The adhering to financial disaster listings in reality the diverse finest herbal herbs for this disorder.

Functioning together with a doctor that recognize dripping digestive tract illness is the very extremely good method you can pick out out.

An extra technique of supplementing your diet plan in addition to supply decrease again equilibrium is thru using organic supplements. A lot of those flowers are loaded with nutrients, minerals and moreover phytonutrients that might enhance your fitness and properly-being.

This hint detail benefits a take a look at if you address dripping gut sickness, baseding on absolutely in recent times released take a look at. It seems that those who revel in this hassle and additionally from maximum of the large issues it turns on-- fibromyalgia-- appear prone to a shortage of magnesium.

The majority of all-herbal health and health experts endorse quantities in among 50 to eighty mg each day. This array is large sufficient, they united states of america, to rebalance any sort of scarcity of zinc. While normally even extra is lots higher, they likewise recommend no longer to take more than a hundred mg a day.

Healthcare professionals likewise propose taking zinc combined with copper. For each 15 mg of zinc you take, you want to take 1 mg of copper. Taking zinc nutritional dietary dietary supplements may additionally additionally need to in truth exhaust your copper degree.

Because the hassle isn't truely really a problem of intake, however absorption, you might be experiencing a lack of magnesium, however the fact that you're consuming components bountiful within the nutrient.

That's why it's miles critical that the swelling is dealt with as promptly as feasible.

Pick your nutritional nutritional supplements very carefully. You want to no longer in reality educate your healthcare provider which you're taking those nutritional dietary supplements, but request insight. She or he recognizes your nice signs and symptoms in addition to has in truth run blood examinations that would make clean exactly what nutrients you lack.

The accessibility of numerous styles of weight-reduction plan A are severa from properly being food establishments, food plan stores, and additionally grocery store stores. If there had been ever earlier than a "superhero" of the vitamins globe, it might absolutely be vitamins C. Some properly-being experts advise as an lousy lot as 4,500 mg of vitamins C ordinary. In some cases taking large portions of vitamin C want to backfire on you and moreover motive digestive machine issues.

This scarcity occurs, partially, whilst your digestive tract wall surfaces grow to be angry, bad a whole lot of the issuer organisation healthful proteins critical for the transport of this mineral.

Taking zinc nutritional supplements, also if your weight loss plan routine is large in substances considerable in this mineral, is a clever concept. Your bodily body uses zinc at a extraordinary rate, so it might be hard to keep tune of its deficiency. It's not unusual that check achieved without a doubt presently by manner of Dr. Keith Eaton, reaping advantages a organisation called Biolab based in London, positioned that zinc is one of the most regular nutritional scarcity among dripping gut illness sufferers.

Chapter 6: Rebalancing With Natural Herbs

It certainly makes feeling that to help recover your leaking intestine disorder, you may in all likelihood preference to transform to those high-quality dietary all-natural permits.

Unsafe elm.

For dripping digestive tract.

Prior to you start any sort of nutritional supplements software, make sure you talk on your person medical expert. Inform her or him exactly what you're making equipped to require to ensure there aren't any troubles with any kind of prescribed drugs you are taking.

If you go to all aware of natural solutions, after that you could currently recognize some component regarding the natural herb volatile elm. For greater than a hundred years, professional herbalists have counted in this plant as a healing salve for injuries, burns, pores and skin swelling, boils, abscess ... Requirement I take place?

An herbalist has simply invested years studying natural herbs with an authorized enterprise. He or she will genuinely be able to help you decide exactly honestly what will surely useful resource your signs and symptoms and signs and symptoms and symptoms and signs and symptoms and symptoms and moreover hassle.

It likewise occurs to be an green representative whilst taken internal. Along with its capacity to deal with coughings, aching throats, as well as looseness of the bowels, this practical herbal herb ought to likewise assist repair tummy problems.

It can also moreover want to amaze you to find out that a number of the pharmaceuticals that hundreds of people depend on in recent times were initially extracted from vegetation. Pain killers and furthermore some coronary coronary coronary heart medicines are honestly 2 archetypes.

Healing with natural herbs is an antique similarly to identified custom further to probable a dependable approach to enhance your nicely-being. A tremendous fashion of societies have in reality depended on vegetation to useful resource them supply decrease again fitness.

Naturally, at the same time as you're trying to find advice from an herbalist, you may wind up with a tick list of suggestions. In the inside the interim, right right right here are some recommendations to collect you considering truly what is feasible.

Why?

Unsafe elm has a mucilage. Mucilage is a material that is primarily based on gel on the same time as combineded with water. It develops a layer and furthermore calms your mouth, throat, belly, further to bowels.

In numerous occasions, the black walnut dietary dietary dietary supplements positioned in diet stores and also natural food stores are made with the hull after it has virtually transformed black. You may intend to labor cautiously with a consultant authorized herbalist with a purpose to guarantee your black walnut strong works.

No, marshmallow starting area.

Has clearly now not whatever to do with s'mores!

When I talk regarding the black walnut green stable, I'm referring to using the inexperienced hull that borders the nut of the black walnut tree. It's critical that the hull is made use of whilst it's miles surroundings-quality.

Consider it for an also a minute and additionally you can concur that pepper mint tea appears to be an organic choice in assisting to alleviate your dripping intestine. Which's because of the truth that herbalists have surely been making use of it for a number of belly issues and additionally other form of problems for ... Nicely, it looks like for lifestyles.

For numerous herbalists, Echinacea is the the the the front runner inside the treatment of Yeast infection on the side of numerous severa exclusive infections.

Goldenseal has in reality the awesome combination of skills that might make it an crucial nutritional complement if you're afflicted with a dripping digestive tract. It not really labors suddenly on digestion worries, however it likewise has anti-bacterial tendencies. In short, it's an natural antibiotic.

The comfort of.

Chamomile tea.

It's enchantment isn't always unexpected thinking about that studies examine validates its overall performance. Numerous studies studies expose that its active components decorate the body immune tool, lower swelling, in addition to has antioxidant top talents.

One extra fave of herbalists inside the remedy of leaking digestive tract is goldenseal, a herbal herb that, like Echinacea has a famous track document whilst it entails digestion issues.

While the herbal herb marshmallow starting has sincerely now not something to do with that delicious campfire praise s'mores, it has each little trouble to do with enjoyable the inflamed mucous membrane layers of your top respiratory tool as well as your digestion device.

If you are now not familiar with Echinacea, you stay in for a thrilling surprise.

Echinacea is one of the maximum typically applied natural herbs on this united states, similarly to with extremely good element. Indigenous Americans utilized it to cope with infections and moreover accidents.

While it might be hard to locate this supplement at your neighborhood meals save, you want to don't have any trouble finding it at herbal meals stores further to weight loss plan shops. And additionally without a doubt, if you can't find out it any form of location else, you may normally collect it online.

This first rate beverage has soothing further to numbing powers. Past that, pepper mint tea gets rid of specific varieties of germs. Also studies take a look at is presently revealing that it is a legitimate safety in desire to acid indigestion further to cranky bowel illness.

Basically, risky elm calms and moreover soothes a swollen in addition to broken digestive tract lining. Particularly, it's miles this calming pastime which ultimately lets in the anti-oxidants to execute their jobs.

Utilizing the perfect offering, it gets rid of now not in reality the grown-up bloodsuckers however the eggs. When I chat concerning the black walnut environment-best strong, I'm concerning the usage of the green hull that borders the nut of the black walnut tree. Echinacea is one of the most significantly made use of natural herbs on this kingdom, further to with first-rate problem. You additionally have the choice of the usage of it in some of kinds. If you're fortunate sufficient to have some fresh herbal herbs, you can preference to dry out the start or the plant itself similarly to vicinity it to apply as a tea.

Generally, herbalists advise which you take Echinacea three instances every day for 7 to 10 days an excellent manner to make sure that you get its whole antibiotic benefits.

This exquisite natural herb likewise includes a wealth of anti-oxidants. In precise, this herbal herb soothes inflammatory infections inside the bowel, according the herbalists.

Certainly, this herbal herb will no longer gain all infections, but it aids individuals who often overuse or perhaps misuse antibiotic pills.

It's known as Pau d'arco, a plant belonging to South America. On that particular continent, its past statistics of utilization is huge ranging. It's been made use of to alter pain, hold joint infection away, as well as to cope with swelling.

In addition, this tea is attributed with strong antispasmodic and also anti inflammatory components, which might be green inside the remedy of tummy issues as well as intestinal tract pains.

If you go through in thoughts taking pau d'arco, you have were given got your alternative inside the type you're taking it. From pill computer systems to dried out bark teas and additionally casts, you can find out any individual of those at herbal food and furthermore weight loss program shops. You might possibly furthermore desire to see a expert herbalist that will help you offered a custom-made method to fulfill your one-of-a-type needs.

Natural herbs that put off.

Bloodsuckers.

And additionally that suggests it is probably genuinely the supplement you are looking for to useful useful aid get better leaking digestive tract disease. Marshmallow starting-- severa times called mallow-- has a recovery past history that actually expands hundreds of years in the formerly.

Pepper mint tea,.

Anybody?

Lots of people discover using Echinacea, the professional herbal herb that is an all-natural antibiotic, assists them in staying smooth of the overuse of prescription anti-biotics. As against seeing their scientific professional and moreover loading a prescription, they hold close this herbal herb.

All you have to deal with this, as a depend of truth, is a solitary mug of chamomile tea ordinary. That's truly easy enough!

When you devour this tea, the active factors on this natural herb tranquility the belly and furthermore advertise the pass of bile, a required lively component inside the meals digestion of fat. This makes it feasible for meals to undergo the stomach quicker.

This foundation is extraordinarily reliable in supporting almost all issues related to the swelling of your digestion device. Maybe simply the answer that would resource you do away with dripping gut.

In this ebook, we've certainly evaluated a number of the way to accumulate your bodily body healthful and balanced thru weight loss plan recurring and moreover supplements-- each dietary in addition to herbal.

One greater beaming movie superstar:.

Goldenseal.

This tea can be furnished nearly anywhere. It's no longer surely effectively to be had in herbal food stores and moreover eating regimen stores, but it may be determined and not using a problem in almost any form of grocery store.

Echinacea similarly to.

The elimination of dripping gut!

Echinacea most likely reached its maximum suitable in enchantment in the 18th as well as nineteenth centuries, additionally on this u . S .. With the improvement of prescription anti-biotics, it unexpectedly discolored from the general public. Currently it's far growing a awesome rebirth as people locate the risks of using severe capsules.

A lot extra often in comparison to no longer, this natural herb is coupled with Echinacea to increase an effective complement that now not honestly assists the digestive device tool, however strengthens your immune gadget.

Utilized globally, you may locate unique elements for human beings to connect with this plant. Makes use of encompass handling scarlet excessive temperature, jungle fever, blood poisoning, as well as diphtheria.

The majority of herbal specialists advocate 1 or 2 tablets taken at the least 2 instances a day. Some declare the maximum offering is tablets three times every day. This very last referral is mainly applicable if you have cranky bowel contamination.

You cannot eliminate tension out of your bodily body, but you can find out the awesome strategies to cope with it well. The adhering to financial disaster gives you some recommendations on the brilliant ways to do really that!

One of the most typical imparting is 3 hundred to 500 mg in pill type 3 instances a day. If you are the use of a forged, you can make use of in between half of to I ml multiple times each day.

It furthermore gadgets off reflux pleasure of the nerve closings to your intestinal gadget, which in a few unspecified time in the future cause a upward thrust in mucous secretion. That's a brilliant idea. This upward thrust in production shields your intestinal device from such conditions as abscess in addition to degree of acidity.

Among the blessings of this recuperation combo is its not unusual overall performance on greater than one hundred severa varieties of bloodsuckers. Utilizing the great presenting, it gets rid of now not clearly the grown-up bloodsuckers however the eggs. The casts are black walnut green, wormwood, further to cloves.

Goldenseal is obtainable nearly everywhere-- in herbal meals shops, food regimen stores, or maybe grocery shop. You have your preference in taking the pill type or the tablet range.

If you're making use of a famous strong essence, you may require 2 to three ml of the fluid. As a powdered essence, you could require three hundred mg of the equal vintage powder.

If you put together this combination in your very very own utilising pepper mint you've got definitely improved on your herbal herb out of doors, hire the dried out fallen leaves of the plant. Prepare your tea thru soaking one tsp of the dried out fallen leaves in a mug of boiling water for approximately 10 minutes.

Below's one you.

Might now not have sincerely come across!

Ways to utilize.

Pepper mint tea.

Expanding your very very non-public pepper mint isn't essential because of the fact that this tea is considerably without a hassle available. You need to moreover buy enteric-lined drugs. These are specifically included so the tablet need to undergo the stomach proper into the gut.

The walnut and also wormwood are the herbal herbs that nicely exterminate the grown-up bloodsuckers, even as the 0.33 herbal herb, the cloves solid, receives rid of the eggs.

Just what concerning that numerous unique reason in addition to huge aggravator of dripping digestive tract ailment: anxiety? At mission, at home or business enterprise, at business enterprise, furthermore on your regular experience.

Pressure as well as chill out the mix. For the very fine effects, devour it four or five instances a day in amongst dishes.

It's an advocated remedy for the cramping and also soreness of the bowels associated with short-tempered bowel illness. Furthermore, chamomile tea aids with the extreme gas and moreover bloating of the intestinal tracts.

Exactly how outstanding is that natural herb? It's being made use of at such an incredible charge that it's far presently overharvested.

We chatted earlier regarding the existence of bloodsuckers in numerous humans that experience leaking digestive tract illness. There is a mixture of three herbal casts you may choice to take that might resource you smooth your physical frame of the bloodsuckers.

Since I actually have it,.

Exactly what do I cease with it?

An greater awesome and additionally substantially made use of tea that might income you is chamomile tea. This tea is currently considered a relaxing and furthermore strain-unfastened dealer; loads of human beings consume it as element in their midnight going to mattress dependancy.

Pau d'arco is usually made use of to address Yeast infections and furthermore any form of form of microbial infections. You're presently aware that Yeast is a situation that is going together with leaking intestine. This herbal herb likewise movements an extra signal of dripping intestine-- the life of bloodsuckers.

Chapter 7: On The Course To Healthiness

Anxiety Administration

and additionally Beyond

Stroll to the lunchroom to speak so an man or woman. Hell, virtually skip down the hall to talk with the assistant.

Several of the most effective individuals attain the maximum excruciating jobs out of the way as rapid as possible. Because approach, they in fact gain them completed in addition to do no longer have time to ... Tension regarding it! And also, maximum appreciably, the jobs do no longer stick round on tomorrow.

Currently, permit's take a look at out some of the physical symptoms and signs and symptoms and signs and symptoms and symptoms and signs and symptoms of a confused physical body. We currently select out that tension need to in the end produce or at least get worse dripping digestive tract contamination. There are severa numerous other indicators:.

It absolutely provided our forefathers properly. The neanderthal skilled anxiety at the equal time as faced with threats which consist of the visibility of a woolly massive. As speedy because the tension system began out, it supplied our historic forefather the sturdiness further to strength every to get rid of the huge animal or to range from it.

A lot extra as compared to that, tension has clearly ended up being one of the motives of unwell fitness and properly being. Did you understand that the Globe Health and nicely-being Company has furnished on-the-manner tension as one of the main 10 factors for lousy fitness and health?

Breathe in sufficient breath that your reduced belly location increases further to drops. Breathe out regularly as you count number to ten.

Several urge tension is an notable thing. And also there are the ones human beings that united states of the us they hard paintings most superb beneath anxiety.

To obtain some jobs, you absolutely require time on my own. I can not talk this hobby with any man or woman else. I do now not invest all my time on my own.

You need to outsmart this remarks through calling a quick day out to do an evaluation of your bodily frame. Some people in truth hold their breath with out also records it.

This is actual when you have actually defended in your private in your place of business seeking to make a due date. Also at the equal time as laboring versus this form of tension, you require to take a periodic damage.

When do I start.

My strain-discount software?

Begin through making an affordable regular for the day earlier. Consist of in this timetable time for strain-discount exercising physical games.

When do you start? Quickly, without a doubt. Initially, you require to do a whole evaluation of your life to see if anxiety is impacting you.

Rather than allowing this chain of sports activities to run its software program software, you may save you it useless in its tracks ... With some method. Take a min-- of direction, I recommend One Minute-- to lessen in addition to take a breath deeply.

Numerous humans try and take treatment of all their desires at even as. You in reality enjoy-- in addition to likely appropriately so-- as if you have truly performed really not anything crucial.

The what is what is that over-committing is some of the giant assets of tension. Rather than regurgitating your arms, clarifying

"That's actually exactly how lifestyles is," intention to address a while.

Are you having hassle identifying? Or maybe you've got had been given in reality positioned you're absent-minded. Various special signs and signs that anxiety can be hurting you absolutely (as well as psychologically) include an obsession with the future, restarting the correct identical thoughts over and over, and additionally the everyday anxiety of failing.

Exercise time manipulate.

Now you in all likelihood understand that thinking about which you can not prevent it, you after that should discover how you may deal with tension as it need to be. You need to unknown wherein to start. Beginning with tiny easy movements further to I assure you'll ultimately experience it in a huge technique.

Numerous independent experts laboring from residence take a day or some of hrs from the day to strolling from a coffeehouse or series.

This is a healthful and balanced habitual. It keeps them associated with others.

Allow's stumble upon it, we can't prevent anxiety. No remember of exactly how hard we strive (or exactly how worried out we collect trying to prevent anxiety), it's far a component of our lives.

Just how pretty a few your day is beginning from go to to go to, consuming at the run, after that hurrying residence in the night time to revel in the very identical exercising exercises simply with numerous locations and moreover objectives?

Indications, indicators ...

Almost everywhere are signs and symptoms and signs!

Just attempt one product at a time. Just cope with one paintings at a time.

Your reaction to anxiety varies from your colleague's. The physical signs and symptoms and signs and symptoms and symptoms and signs and signs and symptoms you create won't be the right identical as each person else's.

The following reaction is generally the arrival of a migraine. At the enormously the very least, you begin to simply feel additionally masses greater distressed.

Yet, you continue to function this method. Rather, strive a numerous approach. Make a list (sure, I apprehend you have definitely completed this within the past, but undergo with me) of all the sports sports that come upon you for that day.

You is probably lured to set up conferences decrease returned to decrease lower back with little if any form of time in between. That way you're now not walking in the back of, emphasized thinking about which you're overdue for the subsequent occasion.

- Belly distress.

- Fast respiration.

- Beating of the heart.

- Limited muscle groups.

- Cold or sweaty arms.

- Migraines.

- Inexplicable exhaustion.

- Rest problems.

- Neck or decrease back troubles.

- Dry mouth.

Are you instantly quick-tempered with pals or relative? This is commonly a number of the very first signs that you're no longer managing tension noticeably nicely.

The first actual time you do that you may count on it is now not laboring. This is a great technique, and furthermore it is a technique you need to discover simply the way to do.

Prior to I talk approximately lasting alternatives along with yoga exercising, exercising (sorry to element out a dirty word), in addition to reflected picture, underneath are couple of moves you can take brief to beneficial useful resource lower your tension diploma.

It ought to take you some of efforts to recognize this. You have to want to make a few changes or additionally take away one or 2 merchandise out of your habitual regularly.

Responding to.

Anxiety.

When you are in individual with a stressful situation, one of the very first bodily signs and symptoms and signs is superficial respiratory. Paradoxically, this feedback surely produces even more tension!

Note the subjects in line with their price. Attempt to apprehend pinnacle priorities. We all have various factors for placing unique sports activities off.

In historical instances, our antique forefathers without a doubt did no longer address tension on a every day or moreover consistent with hour basis, as we do these days. They got here at some stage in tension plenty an awful lot much less usually. The neanderthal's reaction to tension in reality modified right into a life-saving machine in preference to the fitness-draining reaction it has really become.

The what's what's that, in case you permit it, anxiety ought to take a ruining toll in your bodily body. Your response to anxiety may be the numerous motives for leaking intestine ailment.

It simply is one of the ordinary troubles of the twenty first century. Today, you're possibly definitely feeling the anxiety hundreds extra in evaluation to ever in advance than. Anxiety has honestly become an overlooked yet everywhere truth of life.

There are severa one-of-a-kind tiny signs and symptoms and signs, along with nerve-racking laughing or tooth grinding or mandible clenching. And moreover others discover while anxiety is detrimentally influencing them they in truth are masses greater mishap inclined!

Assured, there's a hard and fast of indicators that propose the condition is impacting your physical body. I virtually have clearly unique numerous of them indexed below.

Just the manner you select out to answer to tension affects the circumstance of your properly-being. For beginners, it's far famous that extended direct publicity to stress must in truth reduce your body immune gadget!

Some people manage tension by way of way of resorting to liquor. Has there been a amendment in the amount of cash you eat in a day? You have to likewise find out you're occupying smoking all another time, or when you have sincerely by no means ever surrender, you're smoking greater than commonplace.

One hobby every time.

Today, our reaction to strained situations, to the strain of undertaking, residence, cash, or some aspect else, is reflected in our bodily health. That's proper-- your response to the strain of lifestyles has a immediately bearing in your frame.

As well as this list definitely touches the idea of the iceberg. Also from this, you could see exactly how included your highbrow and additionally bodily fitness and well being is.

Allow me flow one motion furthermore. Researches disclose that taking superb movements-- starting particular programs-- in truth create physical as well as chemical modifications to your physical body that useful resource you to actually feel a long way higher.

Take an extended,.

Deep breath!

Not one humans invests a day without experiencing a few form of tough circumstance. It can be artwork-triggered, or brought on through the difficulty of agreement of fees or a super-tight everyday. Tension is inevitable.

Are you truely feeling nervous, cranky, disturbing? Also surely feeling inexplicable disgrace may want to all be related to a mental remarks to anxiety.

Probably you are experiencing them but not recognizing the source. Also in case you cope with it nutritionally, you may find out it repeats if tension is congesting your lifestyles.

If you are responding inadequately to anxiety, it in truth will expose itself for your moves. Have you decided a alternate in your healthful ingesting practices-- each eating even more or right away having no cravings?

When you're "compelled-out," it's miles verified for your thoughts. You want to discover you are masses extra essential of to your non-public, or you may have determined you certainly can not hobby.

Talk!

Or maybe you may virtually in reality sense a bargain more comfy, at the very least at the start, with composing your troubles out. Merely making your issues or your choices on paper should lay them out as regardless of the reality that an answer sticks out right into your head.

This pointer is an effect to the ultimate one. Among the elements for tension is the failure to speak to all people regarding your method ... Your issues ... Your problems. Also discussing the exquisite events of your lifestyles aids to relieve anxiety.

Remember to snicker!

Are you snug.

Literally?

Once more, this is not definitely an ornate subject. In order to hold tension away, gown as without issues as you may internal your enterprise corporation's robe code. I'm not helping journeying function in pants in addition to a baggie custom t-blouse in case your employees member outlaws this type of clothes.

Past that, ensure your chair suits which the temperature level is within a specific at ease range. Do now not wait up until your putting in the end sooner or later ends up being unbearable to create changes! Being honestly snug minimizes your tension greater than you could photo.

It's regarding time you do. Take a minute to close your eyes. Currently, be aware about all of the data of this vicinity.

No, this isn't always genuinely consisted of as a second idea. Possibly the Visitor's Digest editorial division has sincerely been right the whole time with their pillar, "Giggling is the only treatment." If it is now not the best treatment, it without a doubt charges high up there with the number one 2 or three!

When a hard state of affairs is located inside the the front of you, ask to your very non-public this problem first of all: "Is this honestly my hassle?" It you respond to no, after that forget about it.

A lot more in evaluation to that, tension has in fact emerge as one of the belongings of sick properly being. Did you apprehend that the Globe Wellness Company has sure on-the-procedure tension as one of the essential 10 elements for insufficient health and nicely being? One in three grownups undergo from modest to intense anxiety. In ancient times, our antique forefathers definitely did not address tension on an ordinary or additionally consistent with hour basis, as we do these days. One of the elements for tension is the lack of capacity to talk to any person regarding your interest ... Your issues ... Your issues.

Regardless of what takes place purpose to maintain your funny bone. Find out virtually how now not to absorb your personal as nicely significantly. As nicely as most importantly, find out the great tactics to make fun of in your private.

Determine any shape of movements you may take right away to repair it. Do no longer try to second assumption on your personal.

Can no longer do that by using way of way of your self? You may also intend to buy a CD of directed pictures workout sports.

This isn't always really simply a few arbitrary usage of your creativity. Study currently exhibits that imagining a non violent scene should truly improve you out of your difficult scenario.

Recognize your policies.

Some human beings lose their time in a useless try to modify activities or-- additionally worse-- numerous particular people in order to complete their desires. This in no manner ever labors.

The one-minute getaway.

Do now not limit in your personal needlessly. If you're ladies and additionally want to region on outfit footwears, you may preference to pick out degree ones in choice to heels.

Steven Covey said it perfect in his 7 Routines of Highly Effective Individuals even as he informed us to apprehend just what we need to alter in addition to just what we can not. Concentrate on those topics we have have been given manipulate over!

Do no longer hesitate to jeopardize

You must stay smooth of undesirable tension via the usage of discovering precisely the way to jeopardize. Numerous people advantage dismayed and additionally concerned out whilst any person acts numerous unique they think they need to.

These are movements you could take this exceedingly minute to your normal sports. Right right here are special responsibilities you could begin nowadays-- or in the near future.

Ever before attempted yoga workout?

Remarkably, the phrase yoga exercising comes from the suitable same basis because the phrase yoke. Yoga workout, in an incredibly authentic technique, does genuinely that.

A quantity of the techniques made use of nowadays-- awesome from this vintage method-- are in fact obtained first of all from this project. They embody regulated breathing and moreover meditated photo, psychological pix, and additionally extending similarly to bodily movement.

Lots of human beings employ yoga workout as a way of development, however even more compared to that, its attraction might be credited to its performance in tension management and additionally boosting your bodily health.

Also some groups certainly supply yoga exercise to their personnel individuals. Rather of handling their anxiety, those personnel individuals are traumatic handling the records of their works.

For the lengthiest time, this strain-busting approach had not been recognized inside the Western globe regardless of its famend past facts inside the East. Yoga exercise is a way that dates again not less than five,000 years. It is, absolutely, the earliest shape of self-improvement.

Exactly what

Can yoga exercising do?

You would possibly surely be stunned at the tremendous strain-good deal impacts in addition to bodily benefits of this moderate challenge. A few of yoga exercising's blessings embody:

Generally, yoga workout is the extending of the physical frame proper into diverse gives. At the proper equal time, you're taking a breath regularly and moreover in a regulated manner. Actually, your bodily body now not definitely recognizes an all-herbal country of enjoyment, however it's miles moreover inspired on the very identical time.

Prior to you moreover may also start to obtain as actual with that detail of yoga exercising is bending to your non-public like a cracker, permit me establish you right away. The movements are sincere but very impact at soothing tension.

- Decrease of anxiety

- Decrease of cortisol stages

- Allergic reaction sign consolation

- Slower coronary coronary heart fee

- Decrease in pressure and anxiety

- Boosted stamina

- Bronchial bronchial bronchial bronchial asthma sign relief

- Enhanced resting sports

- Boosted adaptability

- Decline in immoderate blood pressure

- Decrease in muscular tissue stress

- Slowing down of the getting old approach

When you begin locating out a yoga exercise route, you could discover that there are various types of yoga exercise. Some strategies have desires that target religious development, others truly intend to help you decrease anxiety. When you search for a route, ensure to invite precisely what type of yoga exercise the course consists of and moreover the awesome purpose of it.

If you are surfing mainly for a design that decreases your anxiety without a religious ramifications, you are maximum likely searching for a Hatha yoga exercise path.

The effects commonly aren't simply concerned on your head. Current studies study verifies that your physique moreover undertakes a makeover. As you exercising yoga workout, your physical frame launches excessive levels of a chemical known as serotonin, a compound that motives sensations of fitness.

If you want locating out yoga exercise, you may discover a direction near you for individualized hobby. There are numerous DVDs and also guides with out a trouble to be had with a purpose to truly show you the numerous gives.

You do no longer have to

Be a Yogi to exercising meditation

Knowledge? Running off to a cavern might also need to appear appealing at the same time as you are barraged with a myriad of anxieties, it's far as a substitute unwise. When you come from that cold, moist cavern, the strain you left in the back of are probable however going to already current!

It holds authentic that loads of years in advance, pondered image come to be as brief as constrained to the worlds of the non secular elite. Usually, the word reflected photograph summons a photo of a Buddhist monk in a cavern considering the importance of life. Among the handiest understood of these monks is Milarepa, that invested years separated in a supply in the hills of Tibet searching out expertise.

The correct news is, you do now not require to be a Yogi to slight. A Yogi is a player of such eastern faiths as Buddhism, Hinduism, in addition to Taoism that strategies the vintage amazing artwork of contemplated photo.

No, to enjoy the actual advantages of arbitration, you do not have to check in for any shape of spiritual beliefs or likely have any form of need to search for a non secular plateau.

Not remarkably, reflection is rooted in the technique of yoga exercise. Reflection, plenty of people are finding, is an powerful entertainment tool.

Reflection:

Straightforward and additionally fee-effective

That's simply best a tiny-- however crucial-- issue of the power of contemplated picture.

There are on foot reflections. There's a technique of this super paintings which you do while you stroll via a massive maze. (Simply make certain you are not the character supplying the discussion.

The highbrow blessings of this antique method encompass:.

- Rest issues.

- Hypertension.

- Liquor misuse.

- Substance abuse.

- Discomfort.

- Binge consuming.

- Cardiovascular ailment.

- Allergic reactions.

- Anxiousness.

- Cancer cells.

- Bronchial allergies.

- Anxiety.

- Tiredness.

If you're however reluctant because of the truth which you take delivery of as true with you could need to curl your legs pretzel-like proper into the undying, however uncomfortable-appearance whole lotus location, do now not strain. You do now not. (I'm now not honestly fantastic why every yoga exercising and moreover mirrored picture encompass such uneasy poses!).

Corresponding remedy is any kind of valuable help you carry out on the side of traditional treatment. For you, as a affected person of leaking intestine ailment, it does not propose you leave your elimination weight loss program ordinary or your numerous one-of-a-kind treatment plans. It genuinely implies which you exercise meditation together with every numerous special treatment.

Not just that, however it's miles furthermore in fee of round 60 percent of all art work environment crashes and additionally genuinely 30 percentage of every brief- in addition to lengthy-lasting handicaps.

- Knowing to pay hobby on these days minute.

- Watching your disturbing sports from a severa factor of view.

- Boosting a recognition of for your private.

- Developing a easy strain-control program.

- Lowering negative emotions.

Many humans however have the wrong thought that doing away with your mind similarly to enjoyable-- this is all this is-- is some hocus-pocus magic approach. It isn't always honestly. A lot more and moreover an lousy lot greater it's far coming to be a recognized thoughts-body corresponding medicine, diagnosed also via way of allopathic scientific docs.

Modern studies look at is additionally exposing that this approach have to really enhance unique medical issues. Along with supporting you overcome dripping intestine sickness, it has genuinely been understood to assist a large preference of contamination, along with:.

Is reflected picture some.

Hocus-pocus technique?

The most effective facet of contemplated image is that its fantastic non violent cease end result does not stop when you have truly finished your reflected photo session. This honest consultation-- which lasts at the very least 15 or 20 minutes-- ought to useful useful resource you are taking on the the rest of day irrespective of everything's tossed at you!

Think it or not, scientists at Harvard College charge quote that strain payments for fifty to ninety percent of all medical medical doctor's gos to. (Well, likely you, when you have surely seen your scientific professional in recent times with grievances of it.).

Reflection-- as fast as you come to be being acquainted with it-- is simple to carry out and additionally maximum within your finances. It does no longer name for any form of specific devices, regardless of the truth that a few human beings buy calming songs to help them get on the reflective nation.

Much of this tension is associated with our method. Anxiety is stated for without a doubt 20 percent of all the absence within the office.

Just how normally are you preoccupied with exactly what came about in the preceding or the "precisely what ifs" of the future. Reflection makings you right now within the existing-- where all is tranquil!

This sort of pressure-bargain jobs considering that it takes your body right into an stepped forward kingdom of amusement as well as it relaxes your thoughts. Your goal is to get rid of from your thoughts that cluttered movement of mind that are competing collectively with your human mind. When you can obtain this state you may be simply excited with simply exactly how extraordinary you without a doubt sense!

No, you are not the simplest one in case you're virtually feeling the cutting-edge strain of tension, presently are you?

Just how mirrored photo assists!

Not quite, meditated photograph is rooted within the approach of yoga exercise. Reflection, numerous people are locating, is an effective amusement device. A Yogi is a player of such jap faiths as Buddhism, Hinduism, further to Taoism that strategies the old superb art work of mirrored image.

Enter.

Reflection.

Area. You require to look for out a silent area. If you choice songs, make use of a few this is advised for this method.

There's mindfulness reflected image, this is primarily based on. Nicely, being conscious. It's certainly the whole lot about enhancing your recognition and moreover your approval of living in the minute.

It's hard to workout meditation proper after system on the equal time as your thoughts stays competing. You'll discover that it's a awesome deal a lot less tough to get rid of your mind.

As you attention for your respiration, intention to establish all diverse wonderful thoughts apart. If a hassle flip up for your reasoning, delicately aggregate it away. Continuously popularity on your breath.

You're well to your approach to coming across the vintage healing remarkable paintings of mirrored image. You'll be astonished precisely how right away this could alter your aspect of view. You'll likewise be thrilled as you see the anxieties of the day are plenty a whole lot much less right to zap your power.

Pick your type.

Of mirrored image.

There typically aren't loads of tips on this technique, however without a doubt regarding all experts concur: mild with a straight away another time. Some humans exist down all through their reflected photograph.

Sit silently, soothe your mind, and moreover resource to get better your physical body. Study is discovering some unexpected outcomes.

Qi gong is a an vintage Chinese recovery further to electricity exercise. In Chinese, your lifestyles electricity is called Qi or Chi.

Numerous people discover a course and also are led through using a pinnacle degree view or a specific educator after they employ this method. You need to likewise circulate browsing in addition to drift led arbitration lessons.

You ought to begin a honest arbitration approach right presently. Of software, if you make a decision to boom further right into this approach, you may choice to take a direction for you to exercising meditation with others.

As well as do no longer be involved that truly considering which you can not cast off your mind clearly before the whole thing which you're not getting any kind of recuperation advantages. Due to the fact which you are.

It's one of the very first fitness issues that present day studies check recognized may be aided with reflective techniques. It's mainly useful to people that have moderately excessive blood pressure.

In this type, you concentrate your interest on just what you enjoy for the duration of your pondered photograph consultation. Or in desire to removing your thoughts of thoughts, word the thoughts further to feelings.

Breathing is the trick. Think it or otherwise, definitely how we take a breath influences our mind. Among the techniques to green mirrored image is to awareness to your breathing.

Get hold of a rule.

And moreover workout meditation!

To be most green, utilization as numerous detects as feasible. Visualize now not surely the aesthetic cycle, filling up in as hundreds of records as you may, but try to fragrance the sea air if you're visualizing a shoreline.

This, basically, is one of the first-class element of mirrored image. You must be absolutely privy to your respiration. Numerous humans photograph they're taking in peace as they breathe in.

In one more expert research, those humans with chronic ache confirmed a decrease of honestly HALF of their symptoms through mirrored image. That's an amazing final results, but the adhering to attempting to find is lots extra outstanding. This lower lasted for some around 4 years complying with the primary reflected photo education.

(I'm now not in reality tremendous why each yoga exercise and additionally mirrored photograph consist of such awkward poses!).

There are numerous forms of reflected image? That's one of the elegances of this method.

There are though 2 even extra styles of mirrored image, every of these which incorporates bodily hobby. The first actual is Qi gong. Along with reflection as well as bodily movement, it moreover entails executing respiratory exercising exercises.

This method not actually brings approximately tons better health and also energy, baseding on supporters, yet it additionally generates a non violent thoughts-set. Equally as with severa exclusive varieties of reflected photograph, have a have a observe well-known that Qi gong need to help a enormous range of fitness trouble. These embody bronchial bronchial bronchial bronchial asthma, fibromyalgia, joint irritation, migraines, soreness, maximum cancers cells, persistent exhaustion, coronary heart assault, further to most cancers cells.

Among one of the most fantastic manner to workout meditation is through a technique referred to as directed mirrored photo, or led photos or visualization. With this type, you increase intellectual photos of places or notable situations which you find out fun.

Right here's a huge tip: soothing your thoughts completely will now not arise on your very first try. You might probable find to your very personal disturbing casting off thoughts that slip proper into your mind. Ultimately, with true sufficient education, doing away with your mind will absolutely turn out to be much less complicated.

There are countless diverse different research research on the scientific advantages of reflected image. Much an entire lot of to mention proper right right here. You acquire the idea.

Or in case you're loads greater religious, you could preference to duplicate a phrase or expression you discover as element of your non secular method. Lots of usage "shalom.".

Simply as with severa different sorts of reflected picture, have a study well-known that Qi gong have to assist a vast shape of fitness and nicely being troubles.

Relaxing the mind:.

It will now not take location over night time!

Surefire stress-buster:

Workout!

Allow's start with the phrase endorphins. Workout will boom the producing of endorphins.

Workout not truely de-stresses you, but it enhances your well-being. Exactly what you couldn't have definitely recognized is that an extended manner higher health can also need that will help you gather through your day.

All people appear to be that. Our preliminary impulses-- further to inmost need-- in this activities isn't always certainly usually exactly what is greatest for us. Actually, we might in reality all simply sense better if we might honestly carry out a touch workout.

When you relaxation a notable deal better, you could locate you sincerely revel in plenty plenty much less anxiety. As properly as it is able to offer you a revived command over your physical body-- and additionally your existence!

Do you have problem resting at some point of the night time time, thrashing? Does your thoughts pick now not to shut down, going via the day's events in addition to day after present day? Attempt a few workout and additionally you can see that those sleep deprived evenings are reminiscence.

Take a while to exercising, moreover some issue as fundamental as a stroll. You do now not also must take an energetic walk to revel in a far better state of mind. The following time you come house from approach offer it a shot.

Several human beings attempt tough to stay clear of workout in any respect charges. After you come back residence from challenge, psychologically in addition to literally worn-out, you simply without a doubt preference to rest down and also kick your ft up.

It's truly the honestly feeling an man or woman obtains whilst masses more endorphins are to your tool. Any form of prolonged bodily project will really offer you the very identical sensation!

At least, sporting out workout assists to ease the anxiety that commonly lines you through the end of the day.

Getting going:

It's much less tough in evaluation to you agree with!

If you've got trouble beginning in addition to enduring a software program program, reflect onconsideration on getting the help of a friend. Allot time for every of you to stroll with every numerous distinctive. It can be less tough to hold your session in case you understand someone is resting on a park bench watching for you!

.

Currently you are ready to start your de-stressing software software through physical mission. Provide it a shot.

Deal with dripping digestive tract sickness.

Normally!

Prior to you start any shape of exercising application-- also a primary walking software program-- seek advice from your clinical medical doctor. When to procure the inexperienced light from your medical expert, after that you could begin your logo-new existence!

Congratulations! While this manual materials you with the favored devices to start a recuperation software, you have got definitely simply absolutely started out out your quest decrease decrease again to durable, health.

As properly as you could in reality discover that even as you figure out with a close to friend, you are plenty extra determined similarly to a exquisite deal more devoted.

You may be attracted to leap right right into a exercise application all of sudden in addition to without a doubt. It's thoroughly, but, to begin step by step.

Take some time to exercising, moreover some element as honest as a walk. Prior to you start any kind of exercise utility-- also a sincere taking walks ordinary-- seek advice from your medical expert. Workout is exercising. Hell, moreover time invested within the outdoor adoringly regularly tending in your plants can be workout enough to de-stress you.

Final concept.

As properly because of the reality the splendor of it all, you will see that the symptoms and symptoms and symptoms related to your dripping gut sickness are considerably decreased!

As rapid as you start your application, make it a practice. Do now not blow off your regular session with workout!

Do now not moreover provide it a reservation. If you begin with the ones thoughts and moreover hold strolling from it, there can be surely nothing that could cease you in recovery your leaking digestive tract sickness!

Some people start with one type of project truely to find out they tire of it. Probably exactly what you require to do is find out a 2d form of exercise.

When you obtain all started out, you may choice that revel in-nicely-all-over impact that physical undertaking brings. At a few issue (as well as this is probably difficult to think), your physical body will really will let you understand it requires the undertaking.

If you enjoy it, you've got got were given in reality furthermore uncovered that you can see desire at the cease of the passage. Maybe you have really looked at clinical expert after medical medical doctor, expert similarly to expert, definitely to be knowledgeable that those experts cannot discover a supply for your issues.

If you're out of form, you will possibly have hassle doing additionally this a good deal. With sincerely a hint decision and additionally strength of mind, you'll be able to hard work your method as lots as a half of of hr.

As quick as you bought all started out, you could choice that feel-nicely-all-over impact that physical project brings.

Y.

ou similarly to I are coming to the surrender of our quest finding out about dripping intestine illness. You have sincerely placed out that it's far certainly not anything heaps much less in comparison to a stealth situation, impersonating any form of type of severa other conditions, you have got clearly likewise located that identifying this case may be as an opportunity difficult due to the sneakiness of this disease.

Also exercising at a discounted diploma is some distance higher compared to none. As nicely as you could honestly sense an extended way better despite best a little interest in case your bodily body is not honestly useded to it-- assured!

Possibly you are experiencing fibromyalgia. You're complying with every one among your medical medical doctor's orders, taking the most current-day further to first-rate drugs, but but in reality not something assists. You nonetheless revel in soreness.

A lot extra as compared to that, you presently have gadgets at your disposal further to sources at your command to treat leaking digestive tract sickness commonly, without the decision for of tough prescription drug treatments.

Workout is exercise. Hell, additionally time invested in the backyard adoringly having a dishonest to your flora will be workout enough to de-stress you.

Chapter 8: Probiotics

Probiotics are living microorganisms that, when ingested, provide numerous health benefits.They re usually bacteria, but certain types of yeasts can also function as probiotics. You can get probiotics from supplements, as well as from foods prepared by bacterial fermentation. Probiotic foods include yogurt, kefir, sauerkraut, tempeh and kimchi. Probiotics should not be confused with prebiotics, which are dietary fibers that help feed the friendly bacteria already in your gut.

The idea that bacteria are beneficial can be tough to understand. We take antibiotics to kill harmful bacterial infections and use antibacterial soaps and lotions more than ever. The wrong bacteria in the wrong place can cause problems, but the right bacteria in the right place can have benefits. This is where probiotics come in. Probiotics are live microorganisms that may be able to help prevent and treat some illnesses. Promoting a healthy digestive tract and a healthy immune system are their most widely studied benefits at this time. These are also commonly known as friendly, good, or healthy bacteria. Probiotics can be supplied through foods, beverages, and dietary supplements.

The root of the word probiotic comes from the Greek word pro, meaning "promoting," and biotic, meaning "life." The discovery of probiotics came about in the early 20th century, when Elie Metchnikoff, known as the "father of probiotics," had observed that rural dwellers in Bulgaria lived to very old ages despite extreme poverty and harsh climate. He theorized that health could be enhanced and senility delayed by manipulating the intestinal microbiome with host-friendly bacteria found in sour milk. Since then, research has continued to support his findings along with suggesting even more benefits.

Dozens of different probiotic bacteria offer health benefits.

The most common groups include Lactobacillus and Bifidobacterium. Each group comprises different species, and each species has many strains. Interestingly, different probiotics address different health conditions. Therefore, choosing the right type or types of probiotic is essential.

Some supplements known as broad-spectrum probiotics or multi-probiotics combine different species in the same product. Although the evidence is promising, more research is needed on the health benefits of probiotics.

The Power of Probiotic

Probiotics"! use in the form of supplements is controversial. The FDA has not approved any health claims for probiotics. Most studies accept their positive role in helping with diarrhea caused by the use of antibiotics. Some recent studies also show positive impact of probiotic supplements for sufferers of irritable bowel symptoms, although the mechanism is not clear.

In the meantime, the sale of probiotic supplements is growing to a whooping $2.3

billion in 2010. They are being sold as a cure for just about any type of digestive ailment.

Considering the importance of healthy stomach flora, it would seem that probiotic supplements could not hurt. They are not much different from the regular yoghurt, which our mothers pushed at us after a bout of antibiotics. But, if you decide to add probiotic supplement to your nutrition, consult your doctor first. You might have a condition that is counter-indicated and which would make probiotics bad for you. As with any other supplement, don t self-medicate. Any product that contains active ingredients can be potentially harmful.

How Do They Work

Researchers are trying to figure out exactly how probiotics work. Some of the ways they may keep you healthy:

•When you lose "good" bacteria in your body, for example after you take antibiotics, probiotics can help replace them.

•They can help balance your "good" and "bad" bacteria to keep your body working the way it should.

Types of Probiotics

Many types of bacteria are classified as probiotics. They all have different benefits, but most come from two groups. Ask your doctor about which might best help you.

•Lactobacillus. This may be the most common probiotic. It's the one you'll find in yogurt and other fermented foods. Different strains can help with diarrhea and may help people who can't digest lactose, the sugar in milk.

•Bifidobacterium. You can find it in some dairy products. It may help ease the symptoms of irritable bowel syndrome (IBS) and some other conditions.

•Saccharomyces boulardii is a yeast found in probiotics. It appears to help fight diarrhea and other digestive problems.

What Do They Do

Among other things, probiotics help send food through your gut by affecting nerves that control gut movement. Researchers are still trying to figure out which are best for certain health problems. Some common conditions they treat are:

•Irritable bowel syndrome

•Inflammatory bowel disease (IBD)

•Infectious diarrhea (caused by viruses, bacteria, or parasites)

•Diarrhea caused by antibiotics

There is also some research that shows they're useful for problems in other parts of your body. For example, some people say they have helped with:

•Skin conditions, like eczema

•Urinary and vaginal health

•Preventing allergies and colds

•Oral health

Chapter 9: Importance Of Microorganisms For Your Gut

The complex community of microorganisms in your gut is called the gut flora or microbiota. In fact, your gut contains hundreds of different types of microorganisms as many as 1,000, according to some estimations.This includes bacteria, yeasts and viruses with bacteria making up the vast majority.Most of the gut flora is found in your colon, or large intestine, which is the last part of your digestive tract.

Surprisingly, the metabolic activities of your gut flora resemble those of an organ. For this reason, some scientists refer to the gut flora as the "forgotten organ". Your gut flora performs many functions that are important for health. It manufactures vitamins, including vitamin K and some of the B vitamins.

It also turns fibers into short-chain fats like butyrate, propionate and acetate, which feed your gut wall and perform many metabolic functions. These fats also stimulate your immune system and strengthen your gut wall. This can help prevent unwanted substances from entering your body and provoking an immune response.

However, not all organisms in your gut are friendly.Your gut flora is highly sensitive to your diet, and studies show that an unbalanced gut flora is linked to numerous diseases.These diseases include obesity, type 2 diabetes, metabolic syndrome, heart disease, colorectal cancer, Alzheimer's and depression. Probiotics and prebiotic fibers can help correct this balance, ensuring that your "forgotten organ" is functioning optimally.

Impact on Digestive Health

Probiotics are widely researched for their effects on digestive. Strong evidence suggests that probiotic supplements can help cure antibiotic-associated diarrhea. When people take antibiotics, especially for long periods of time, they often experience diarrhea even long after the infection has been eradicated.

This is because the antibiotics kill many of the natural bacteria in your gut, which shifts gut balance and allows harmful bacteria to thrive.

Probiotics also combat irritable bowel syndrome (IBS), a common digestive disorder, reducing gas, bloating, constipation, diarrhea and other symptoms. Some studies also note benefits against inflammatory bowel diseases, such as Crohn's disease and ulcerative colitis.

What s more, probiotics may fight Helicobacter pylori infections, which are one of the main drivers of ulcers and stomach cancer. If you currently have digestive problems that you can't seem to vanquish, a probiotic supplement may be something to consider   though you should consider consulting with your doctor first.

Impact on Weight Loss

People who are obese have different gut bacteria than those who are lean. Interestingly, animal studies indicate that fecal transplants from lean animals can make obese animals lose weight. Therefore, many scientists believe that your gut bacteria are important in determining body weight. Although more research is needed, some probiotic strains appear to aid weight loss.

In one study in 210 people with central obesity, which is characterized by excess belly fat, taking the probiotic Lactobacillus gasseri daily resulted in an 8.5% loss of belly fat over 12 weeks.

When participants stopped taking the probiotic, they gained the belly fat back within four weeks. Evidence also suggests that Lactobacillus rhamnosus and Bifidobacterium lactis can assist with weight loss and obesity prevention though this needs more research. Conversely, some animal studies demonstrate that other probiotic strains could lead to weight gain, not loss.

Other Health Benefits

There are many other benefits of probiotics. They affect:

•Inflammation: Probiotics reduce systemic inflammation, a leading driver of many diseases.

•Depression and anxiety: The probiotic strains Lactobacillus helveticus and Bifidobacterium longum have been shown to reduce symptoms of anxiety and depression in people with clinical depression.

•Blood cholesterol: Several probiotics have been shown to lower total and bad LDL cholesterol levels.

•Blood pressure: Probiotics may also cause modest reductions in blood pressure.

•Immune function: Several probiotic strains may enhance immune function, possibly leading to a reduced risk of infections, including for the common cold.

•Skin health: There is some evidence that probiotics can be useful for acne, rosacea and eczema, as well as other skin disorders.

This is only a small slice of probiotics total benefits, as ongoing studies indicate a wide breadth of health effects.

Safety and Side Effects

Probiotics are generally well tolerated and considered safe for most people. However, in the first few days, you may experience side effects related to digestion, such as gas and mild abdominal discomfort.

After you adjust, your digestion should begin improving.

In people with compromised immune systems, including those with HIV, AIDS and several other conditions, probiotics can lead to dangerous infections. If you have a medical condition, consult with your doctor before taking a probiotic supplement.

However, probiotic supplements offer a wide range of benefits with few side effects so if you re interested in improving your gut health, they could be worth a shot.

Chapter 10: Leaky Guts

Before the medical community had better understanding of the mechanisms that cause disease, doctors believed certain ailments could originate from imbalances in the stomach. This was called hypochondriasis. (In Ancient Greek, hypochondrium refers to the upper part of the abdomen, the region between the breastbone and the navel.) This concept was rejected as science evolved and, for example, we could look under a microscope and see bacteria, parasites, and viruses. The meaning of the term changed, and for many years, doctors used the word "hypochondriac" to describe a person who has a persistent, often inexplicable fear of having a serious medical illness.

But what if this ancient concept of illnesses originating in the gut actually holds some truth? Could some of the chronic diseases our society faces today actually be associated with a dysfunctional gastrointestinal system?

The expression "leaky gut" is getting a lot of attention in medical blogs and social media lately, but don't be surprised if your doctor does not recognize this term. Leaky gut, also called increased intestinal permeability, is somewhat new and most of the research occurs in basic sciences. However, there is growing interest to develop medications that may be used in patients to combat the effects of this problem.

What exactly is leaky gut

Inside our bellies, we have an extensive intestinal lining covering more than 4,000 square feet of surface area. When working properly, it forms a tight barrier that controls what gets absorbed into the bloodstream. An unhealthy gut lining may have large cracks or holes, allowing partially digested food, toxins, and bugs to penetrate the tissues beneath it. This may trigger inflammation and changes in the gut flora (normal bacteria) that could lead to problems within the digestive tract and beyond. The research world is booming today with studies showing that modifications in the intestinal bacteria and inflammation may play a role in the development of several common chronic diseases.

Who gets a leaky gut (and why)

We all have some degree of leaky gut, as this barrier is not completely impenetrable (and isn't supposed to be!). Some of us may have a genetic predisposition and may be more sensitive to changes in the digestive system, but our DNA is not the only one to blame. Modern life may actually be the main driver of gut inflammation. There is emerging evidence that the standard American diet, which is low in fiber and high in sugar and saturated fats, may initiate this process. Heavy alcohol use and stress also seem to disrupt this balance.

We already know that increased intestinal permeability plays a role in certain gastrointestinal conditions such as celiac disease, Crohn's disease, and irritable bowel syndrome. The biggest question is whether or not a leaky gut may cause problems elsewhere in the body. Some studies show that leaky gut may be associated with other autoimmune diseases (lupus, type 1 diabetes, multiple sclerosis), chronic fatigue syndrome, fibromyalgia, arthritis, allergies, asthma, acne, obesity, and even mental illness. However, we do not yet have clinical studies in humans showing such a cause and effect.

What causes leaky gut

In many cases, leaky gut is caused by your diet. For me, certain foods that I was consuming every day, including gluten, soy and dairy, were being treated by my body as foreign invaders that had to be fought off. When I ate these foods, my body went to war, producing antibodies, which triggered an immune response that included diarrhea, headaches, fatigue and joint pain.

Leaky gut can also be caused by medications including antibiotics, steroids or over-the-counter pain relievers like aspirin and acetaminophen, which can irritate the intestinal lining and damage protective mucus layers. This irritation can start or continue the inflammation cycle that leads to intestinal permeability.

Signs you have a leaky gut

According to Dr. Leo Galland, director of the Foundation for Integrated Medicine, the following symptoms might be signs of leaky gut:

•Chronic diarrhea, constipation, gas or bloating

•Nutritional deficiencies

•Poor immune system

•Headaches, brain fog, memory loss

•Excessive fatigue

•Skin rashes and problems such as acne, eczema or rosacea

•Cravings for sugar or carbs

•Arthritis or joint pain

•Depression, anxiety, ADD, ADHD

•Autoimmune diseases such as rheumatoid arthritis, lupus, celiac disease or Crohn's

•How to heal a leaky gut

The key to healing a leaky gut is changing your diet and eliminating the foods that your body treats as toxic. On the advice of my nutritionist, I eliminated gluten, dairy, soy, refined sugar, caffeine and alcohol. Within six weeks, I was feeling like a new person. My energy levels were way up, the diarrhea and bloating had subsided, and I was sleeping like a baby at night.

In addition to eliminating certain foods, I added a few things to help repair my leaky gut. These included healthy fats such as fish, coconut and olive oils; avocados and flax; probiotics to restore the healthy bacteria in my gastrointestinal tract; and L-glutamine, an amino acid that rejuvenates the lining of the intestinal wall.

Within three months, I had controlled my leaky gut. I have to adhere to my new dietary changes or I suffer the consequences diarrhea, bloating and fatigue. But it's a small price to pay for feeling so alive and healthy again!

If you have any of the symptoms I mentioned, get checked by your health care provider. I had sensitivities to certain foods, but your symptoms could be caused by other issues. It's important to design a treatment plan that fits your issues.

Chapter 11: A Path Toward A Healthier Gut

Although it is unusual to hear the term "increased intestinal permeability" in most doctors' offices, alternative and integrative medicine practitioners have worked on gut healing as an initial step to treat chronic diseases for decades. Other cultures around the world often recommend specific diets to make people feel better. Even in the United States, it is common to see people changing their diets after getting sick. A common initial step some practitioners take is to remove foods that can be inflammatory and could promote changes in the gut flora. Among the most common are alcohol, processed foods, certain medications, and any foods that may cause allergies or sensitivities. In my practice, I often see patients improve significantly when they start eating a healthier diet.

Controversy still exists on whether leaky gut causes the development of diseases outside the gastrointestinal tract in humans. However, it is always a good idea to eat a nutritious, unprocessed diet that includes foods that help quell inflammation (and avoids foods known to trigger inflammation), which may, at least in theory, help to rebuild the gut lining and bring more balance to the gut flora. This recipe could make you feel better, without any side effects. It is definitely worth a try.

Leaky Gut Syndrome

"Leaky gut syndrome" is said to have symptoms including bloating, gas, cramps, food sensitivities, and aches and pains. But it's something of a medical mystery. "Physicians don't know enough about the gut, which is our biggest immune system organ."

"Leaky gut syndrome" isn't a diagnosis taught in medical school. Instead, "leaky gut really means you've got a diagnosis that still needs to be made." "You hope that your doctor is a good-enough Sherlock Holmes, but sometimes it is very hard to make a diagnosis."

"We don't know a lot but we know that it exists," "In the absence of evidence, we don't know what it means or what therapies can directly address it."

Intestinal Permeability

A possible cause of leaky gut is increased intestinal permeability or intestinal hyperpermeability. That could happen when tight junctions in the gut, which control what passes through the lining of the small intestine, don't work properly. That could let substances leak into the bloodstream.

People with celiac disease and Crohn's disease experience this. "Molecules can get across in some cases, such as Crohn's, but we don't know all the causes." Whether hyperpermeability is more of a contributing factor or a conseꟼuence is unclear. But why or how this would happen in someone without those conditions is not clear.

Little is known about other causes of leaky gut that aren't linked to certain types of drugs, radiation therapy, or food allergies.

Unsolved Mystery

Leaky gut symptoms aren't unique. They're shared by other problems, too. And tests often fail to uncover a definite cause of the problem. That can leave people without a diagnosis and, therefore, untreated. It's crucial, to find a doctor who will take time with you and take your concerns seriously. "You may have leaky gut and we may be able to treat what causes it," "If you have something going on, it is incumbent upon the medical community to listen to you."

Unfortunately, Lee says, not all doctors make the effort to get at the root of the problem, and that's what frequently sends patients to alternative practitioners.

"Often, the reason they have resorted to alternative medicine is because of what they have been told and how they have been treated by other practitioners." "We need to listen."

Treatment Without Research

In her clinic, Lee combines conventional medicine with evidenced-based complementary therapies. But with leaky gut, she says, the evidence about what causes it and how to treat it has yet to fully accumulate. This is something that is essential for patients to understand.

"We are in the infancy of understanding what to do." "People who are making claims about what to do are doing so without evidence."

For example, many web sites offering information on leaky gut, recommend taking L-glutamine supplements to strengthen the lining of the small intestine. Theoretically, that makes sense, given glutamine's role in intestinal function but there is no research to back up such claims. "There's no evidence that if I give you a pile of glutamine pills, that you will improve."

Lifestyle May Matter

Treating the underlying condition, such as Crohn's or celiac disease, will often resolve symptoms associated with the condition. But without a firm diagnosis, a doctor's hands are often tied by a lack of evidence. Diet likely plays a big role in having a leaky gut, Lee and Kirby agree. So if you have symptoms of leaky gut, you would do well to see a gastroenterologist who is also trained in nutrition.

Chronic stress may also be a factor. "You need to tend to your stress, whether through medication or meditation. That's what you need to focus on." "Chronic health problems are so often due to lifestyle, and we don't have pills for those." "We're talking about the way we live and the way we eat."

Probiotics and Leaky Gut

A healthy gut is dependent on a high level of probiotics. The risk factors that often lead to leaky gut often cause inflammation and a lack

179

of functioning of the mucous layer that protects the intestinal epithelium. Experts believe that probiotics reduce these risk factors and lower the chances of developing leaky gut.

Probiotics can increase the production of protective cells along the mucosal wall. This increases the health of the gut wall, which makes the selective permeability of the wall work the way it is supposed to work.

Probiotics have also been found to help in the secretion of inflammatory mediators and in the development of the immune system. Probiotics help the immune system develop during critical periods of growth and break down bad bacteria and viruses helping to reduce the risk of allergic diseases.

Chapter 12: Ways Probiotics Actually Help With Leaky Gut

1) Probiotics can support your gut lining's 'gatekeepers' (a.k.a. Tight junctions) This is very important, because your tight junctions are the guys that decide if something should pass through the lining (and into your bloodstream) or not.

When working right, tight junctions will allow molecules which are good (hello nutrients) to get through, whilst it will ensure those that are bad (hello undigested large food particles, toxins etc) stay out. By selectively allowing entry like this you get better nutrient absorption. Which is fantastic. And by preventing toxins slipping through and into the bloodstream, you help to lower unnecessary immunity responses / inflammation. Even better!

2) Probiotics can prevent bad bacteria and yeast from hanging around

Obviously, this means less leaky gut. But it can also help with related conditions like SIBO and candida, respectively. So it's no wonder that I sometimes think of probiotics like mini Gandalfs (from Lord of the Rings) shuttling around your intestines yelling at bad bacteria "Thou shall not pass!".

Unsurprisingly probiotics are being used these days to target bad bacteria in other parts of the body too, including your teeth (eg tooth decay and periodontal disease).

3) Probiotics can help us break down foods and turn them into nutrients

This is a more indirect digestion aid than say digestive enzymes themselves, but very helpful nonetheless. Because as we know, breaking down our food better will reduce the number of large particles bombarding our poor ol intestinal lining.

4) Probiotics have been shown to reduce leaky gut markers!

Best of all, probiotics don't just sound good on paper. Perhaps the coolest thing about them is that recent studies have shown that markers of intestinal permeability decrease dramatically when probiotics are taken!

For example, in this randomized, double-blind and placebo-controlled study, zonulin levels in subjects' feces were "significantly reduced" after 14 weeks of probiotic use compared to those who didn't take probiotics. And since less zonulin means less intestinal permeability, the results indicate probiotics can lead to a healthier intestinal wall.

More ways probiotics work to support your leaky gut

Probiotics can assist in the secretion of inflammatory mediators. Which is kinda like organizing your emergency services so they're all on the same page and not all going around blaring their sirens simultaneously and causing havoc. Probiotics can support secretion of additional intestinal mucus (the protective layer for your gut lining/wall).

Probiotics can even help break down fiber into beneficial short chain fatty acids like butyrate, which your gut absolutely loves.

Eating versus supplementing with probiotics

You see, whilst others out there will just pick a side and argue it into the ground, I'm a big fan of both probiotic foods and supplements. I see them as extremely complementary.

To help you work out what mix of probiotic foods versus supplements, makes sense, I'll run through the pros and cons of each, including showing where each one makes the most sense.

Why I love probiotic foods

•Packed with billions of CFUs – most probiotic foods, eg live sauerkraut, can deliver billions of probiotics with every spoonful. In other words, they can be incredibly potent!